LOVE IN ABUNDANCE

A Counselor's Guide to Open Relationships

By Kathy Labriola

greenery press

Cover design by Hollis Duncan

Published in the United States by Greenery Press, P.O. Box 5280, Eugene, OR 97405, www.greenerypress.com.

Distributed by SCB Distributors, Gardena, CA.

Contents

This book is dedicated to Rick and Eric, who should each receive a Labriola Endurance Medal for sticking with me all these years through all of life's little twists and turns.

PART ONE

Polyamory and Open Relationships — What Are They And How Do They Work?

1 Introduction to Open Relationships and Polyamory

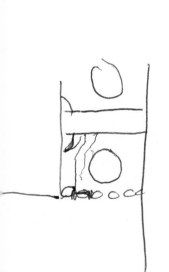

Two terms, "open relationships" and "polyamory," are used almost interchangeably, and can be very confusing. Because these terms are relatively new to the English language, there is little consensus on their exact meanings. In general, both refer to having the freedom to be sexually and/ or emotionally involved with more than one person. While some may quibble about subtle differences in these terms, it doesn't really matter what you call your relationship or lifestyle as long as you are clear with your partner(s) about exactly what you mean. This book uses both terms and considers them identical.

There is a key difference between these arrangements and old-fashioned infidelity or "cheating." Open relationships and polyamorous relationships are explicitly designed to be practiced honestly, with the mutual consent of all parties — where no one is deceived and everyone chooses to enter this type of relationship.

Some people in these types of alternative relationships are married or live with a "primary" lover or spouse, but occasionally have casual sexual relationships outside their marriages. Some have more than one committed long-term relationship concurrently. Others are in "group marriages," living with several adults who share sexual and spousal relationships. Still other people are inclined toward many relationships of a less committed nature, and are not seeking marriage or long-term relationships. Part One of this book will cover the different types of open relationships and the pros and cons of each model.

Many other people embrace the theory of open relationships and enjoy having the option of having more than one lover or spouse if they should desire, but may not have the time or energy for more than one relationship, or may not have met the right person or people to enter into such an arrangement. So even though they consider themselves polyamorous, they may not "practice" polyamory — but they like having the option and having an agreement with their partner that another relationship will be acceptable if it does happen. For many people, having the freedom to choose additional relationships is as important and fulfilling as actually acting on this option and having other lovers.

Relationships outside the monogamous paradigm are nothing new; they have been practiced since the beginning of humankind. However, until recently, polyamory was considered immoral, deviant behavior in most Western cultures, was identified as a major taboo in most religions, and was generally done secretly—"cheating" on one's wife or husband and lying about it, while pretending to be the "faithful" spouse.

Due to sexism and women's economic dependence on men throughout most of history, men could usually get away with extramarital affairs, mistresses, sexual relationships with prostitutes, and even having several wives, because women's powerless economic and political position forced them to accept any and all behavior from their husbands. Women were much less at liberty to stray outside of marriage and have other relationships. This confinement was partly because their primary responsibility for home and children seriously restricted their mobility, partly due to lack of effective birth control methods, and partly because the "adulteress" was usually severely punished by society for her transgression. However, the philandering husband generally was tolerated with a "boys will be boys" attitude.

This double standard continues today in most of the world. However, in Western industrialized nations, we have benefited from the "sexual revolution" of the 1960s and '70s. New freedoms were fueled by the advent of effective birth control methods such as birth control pills, the legalization of abortion, and by women entering the paid labor force and achieving more economic independence from men. This transformation of sexual mores gave both men and women the opportunity to experiment with many new types of relationships and made it possible to reject the rigid sex roles and limitations of monogamous relationships.

Why Do Some People Want More Than One Partner?

No one knows the answer to this question, just as no one knows exactly why some people are gay, others bisexual, and still others are straight. Many people are very happy with monogamous relationships, and believe that a monogamous relationship promises greater security, stability, and protection from HIV and other sexually transmitted infections. Such people may feel more fully loved and feel they can experience deeper intimacy in an exclusive relationship with one person. Or they may feel that monogamy is just simpler and more feasible to fit into their busy lives than more open relationships.

On the other hand, many people try to live a monogamous lifestyle and find it just does not meet their needs. They come to believe that it is unrealistic to expect any one person to fulfill all their needs for intimacy, companionship, love, and sex, for the rest of their lives. Many people practice "serial monogamy"—having one monogamous relationship after another, each one ending due to some area of incompatibility or dissatisfaction. Many people spend their whole life searching for the perfect mate, only to find themselves dissatisfied time after time. They cannot maintain a monogamous relationship over the long haul, because one partner or the other "cheats" and has secret affairs, or one partner loses interest in the other, or one or both partners discover conflicts or incompatible needs. Many people decide to explore more open forms of relationships as a way of avoiding some of the problems they have experienced in monogamous relationships.

What Does This Type of Relationship Offer?

Boiled down to its essence, people are drawn to an open relationship because they want either More or Different. If they are looking for More, it's because they love everything they are getting in their current relationship(s) but are not getting quite enough: "not quite enough" romance, attention, sex, time, or specific activities. So they want to supplement their current relationship by getting some of that missing quantity with someone else.

If, instead, they want Different, they enjoy and value their current relationship, but feel they are missing one or more crucial ingredients that really would make them happier, so they are seeking that "other something" from someone else. For instance, they want a different type of sexual activity ("my partner doesn't like oral sex"), or a partner of a different gender, a person who is more romantic or adventurous, someone with whom they have some specific shared interest ("my partner hates camping and I love it"), or the novelty of sexual and romantic variety with a new or different person.

In addition, many monogamous relationships suffer from excessive dependency. Couples usually live together and spend their free time together, sometimes to the exclusion of all other intimate friendships. Each partner depends heavily on the other for emotional support, socializing, "family," and community. Many people give up friends, social activities, even sports and hobbies if their partner doesn't share an interest in these activities, often creating resentment and dissatisfaction.

Monogamous couples agree to depend solely on each other for affection and sex, and many become dissatisfied due to sexual incompatibilities, differences in level or frequency of sex, or boredom with their sexual patterns. When they feel strong sexual attractions towards others, they must repress these feelings or end their current relationship in order to have sex with someone else. Many complain that although they love their spouse and feel strongly attracted to him or her, the spouse doesn't want sex frequently enough or does not enjoy the same sexual activities. This leaves one partner always wanting more sex or more variety in sexual practices, and the other always feeling pressured for sex, often resulting in one partner having secret affairs with other lovers to fulfill their sexual needs.

Relationships outside monogamy can create solutions for some of these problems. Non-monogamous people have opportunities to become more independent, and often have many friends and many sources of emotional support rather than depending on their spouse for everything. People in open relationships must be assertive and able to articulate their own needs clearly and honestly. Being in non-monogamous relationships offers the opportunity to meet all your needs rather than repress and resent whichever needs do not conveniently fit into your initial relationship. It allows each partner to have as much sex, or as little sex, as he or she wants, because the partner who wants more sex is free to have other sexual relationships. Many basically good relationships end because of sexual incompatibilities or because of excess dependency, and these alternatives can offer a way to continue a good relationship while solving some of these problems. Non-monogamy can strengthen relationships by encouraging each partner to be honest with themselves and each other, and to communicate clearly about feelings, needs, anxieties, and insecurities, including jealousy.

Part Two will discuss the basic "nuts and bolts" of polyamorous relationships and important communication skills, to give you an idea of what you will need to learn to establish successful relationships.

What Are the Problems With Open Relationships?

It is possible for the various types of non-monogamous lifestyles to enrich the lives of all parties involved and lead to deeper intimacy, love, and satisfaction. However, in real life, making a transition from traditional relationships to a non-monogamous lifestyle is very stressful and involves "growing pains," because living in a new way requires learning new skills and overcoming a lifetime of socialization. What sounds idyllic and reasonable in theory may be complicated and difficult to work out in reality — logistically as well as emotionally. People with the best of intentions often discover that they have many intense insecurities and fears based on core beliefs about themselves, about their partner(s), and about relationships and family in general.

Most people find that they experience jealousy to a lesser or greater extent, especially when first embarking on this lifestyle. Managing and mitigating jealousy usually takes time, thought, talking it out, and reassurance from partners. Some people find that while they continue to feel jealous at times and to have feelings of conflict and ambivalence about their lifestyle and relationships, these feelings are greatly outweighed by a much more positive experience of the benefits and freedom of polyamory. Part Three covers different aspects of the "green-eyed monster" and provides many tools for managing jealousy.

After the initial fear of change and the anxiety of charting unknown territory subsides, many people feel comfortable with open relationships as long as they feel secure that they are loved and will not be abandoned. One strategy that has worked well to minimize fears and jealousy is to decide on rules and parameters which feel safe and supportive, and negotiate with your partner(s) to reach agreement on what type of non-monogamous lifestyle best fits your needs.

For instance: Is it okay to have casual affairs? Do you want advance notice if your partner meets someone and wants to initiate a sexual relationship? Does your spouse or partner(s) have veto power over your choice of potential partners? Do you have an agreement on safer-sex guidelines to prevent being exposed to sexually transmitted diseases like syphilis, herpes, gonorrhea, chlamydia, hepatitis, and HIV? Do you want to participate in sexual relationships with more than one partner, or be involved with your partner's lovers? Do you feel you will have enough love and attention from your partner if he or she has other relationships? How much time will you allow your partner to spend with other lovers? Who will spend holidays and vacations together? What about children and other family members — do you want to have children, and who will have parental responsibilities? Will all partners live with you? Is one partner a primary spouse or are all partners equally important in terms of time and commitment? Will you pool your financial resources or do you want financial autonomy? Are you going to "come out" about your lifestyle to family, friends, and co-workers, or would you prefer to keep your relationships private?

While many of these questions need to be addressed in any relationship, they are even more crucial to discuss in non-monogamous relationships, and can go a long way toward preventing misunderstandings, anger, and jealousy. Most people experience less of the anxiety and more of the satisfaction of a polyamorous lifestyle if they know what to expect, and feel secure that their partners will abide by rules that are mutually agreed upon.

Part Four presents some of the tools that will enable you to surive and thrive in an open relationship – from dealing with new relationships intruding on the primary relationship, to managing differing needs for intimacy and autonomy, to establishing the legal paperwork to protect your money, health, possessions, and children. Learning about how others have worked to creatively solve these problems may help you avoid some of the common pitfalls or correct them more easily.

In Part Five, the final chapters of the book address some specialized issues such as polyamorous BDSM relationships, sex addiction, the controversy among feminists over polyamory, and skills for secondary, or "outside," partners.

At the end of the book is a short list of additional resources that can provide more information and education on open relationships. More reading and education is recommended for anyone exploring this exciting and challenging relationship style!

Because each polyamorous situation is as unique as the particular individuals involved, only trial and error will tell what will work for each relationship or family. A lifestyle may look great on paper but may feel completely different "on the ground," and living the lifestyle — with an open mind and some rules that feel comfortable — is the only way to develop a long-term situation that works for everyone involved.

Because openly polyamorous lifestyles are still relatively rare, few role models are available to demonstrate the different kinds of open relationships. Now that you have a basic idea of what open relationships are all about, the next chapter will discuss the three basic types of open relationships that are widely practiced. The advantages and drawbacks of each one will be described to help you decide which, if any, of these models may be feasible for you.

2 Models of Open Relationships

The model of heterosexual, monogamous marriage is sanctioned by society, religion, and the law as the only acceptable type of sexual relationship. In fact, we are so heavily socialized to believe in the ideals of monogamy and marriage that many people cannot even imagine any other option. Frequent responses to the idea of open relationships are: "But I've never seen one"; "No one I know has ever tried that"; and "There's no way it could possibly work out." People often ask, "But how does it work? What's it like?"

In fact, many successful models do exist, and are being practiced at this minute by happy singles, couples and groupings around the world. This chapter will give you an overview of the three main types of non-monogamous relationships and the numerous variations on those models. Before you begin thinking about new ways of living, it can help to see some examples and to understand the advantages and drawbacks of each model. By examining each model, you may be able to discern whether an open relationship is right for you and, if so, which model may best fit your individual lifestyle. The possibilities are limitless and you can "customize" any of these models to accommodate your needs.

The Primary/Secondary Model

This is by far the most commonly practiced form of open relationship and it is the most similar to monogamous marriage. In this model, the "couple relationship" is considered primary, and any other relationships revolve around the couple. It is most frequently practiced by married people or other couples in long-term relationships. The couple decides that their relationship will have precedence over any outside relationships. The couple usually lives together and forms the primary family unit, while other relationships receive less time and priority. No outside relationship is allowed to become equal in importance to the primary relationship. The couple makes the rules; secondary lovers have little power over decisions and are must accept the parameters set by the primary couple.

There are several distinct variations of this mode, including:

a) Heterosexual couples who are "swingers." They attend sex parties or meet sexual partners through personal ads or through various activities and networks. Some couples only have sex with other couples. Others engage in three-way sex by locating another man for the woman or another woman for the man, and only have sexual adventures with their spouse present. Still other swinging couples allow either spouse to have recreational sex with other partners without the spouse present, but as this is strictly casual sex, no emotional involvement or commitment is allowed.

For example:

Jane and Jim are a straight, married couple. They answer personals ads on adult websites and have sex only with other couples, together as a foursome.

Rose and Bill live together. Rose goes to sex parties and has anonymous sex with other men. Bill enjoys meeting women in bars and clubs for casual sex.

b) Gay male couples who go to the baths, the bars, sex clubs, or adult bookstores for recreational and/or anonymous sex. Many gay couples engage in this activity together, or have only "three-ways." Such couples typically have an agreement that either partner can go out alone and have sex with other men, but the goal is casual sex rather than relationships. Some lesbian couples have similar agreements, but this relationship style is much more common among gay men and heterosexuals than lesbians.

For example:

Joe and Jim are a gay male couple who enjoy going to the baths together and meeting younger guys for three-way sex. Joe also likes to go to the park and have anonymous sex with other men, and occasionally answers personal ads to meet casual sex partners.

c) Couples of any and all sexual orientations who allow each spouse to have outside sexual relationships, either casual or long-term. These outside relationships are still considered secondary, and if any conflict develops, the primary couple relationship will take precedence. Usually the couple lives together, shares finances, and spends weekends, holidays, and vacations together. The outside lovers usually do not live with them. They spend much less time together than the primary couple, have very little voice in decisions and rule-making, and must arrange scheduling around the demands of the primary relationship. Some couples have rules that each spouse has "veto power" over any new lovers that his or her spouse may choose: in other words, if a woman is interested in a relationship with a new man, her husband has the power to veto that relationship before it starts. Other couples allow each person to sleep with whomever they choose, but make rules about how much time they can spend with their other lovers, whether they can spend the night away from home, whether they can spend any weekend time with them. Other agreements may include safer sex guidelines and other restrictions.

For example:

Clare and Tom live together. Clare has a long-term sexual relationship with her neighbor, Melissa, who spends a lot of afternoons with Clare while Tom is at work. Tom has a series of short-term relationships with women he meets on-line through polyamorous websites. However, Tom fell in love with one of his outside lovers, so Clare insisted that he break off the relationship because it threatened the primary couple relationship.

Alan and Damon are a gay couple who live together. Alan has two "fuck-buddies," friends he regularly has sex with. Damon has a long-term boyfriend in L.A. whom he sees for a few days each month when he is there on business.

David and Lucy are a bisexual couple who are married and have two children. David has a long-term male lover whom he sees frequently, but he considers his marriage and children his first priority and devotes more time and commitment to them. Lucy has had several female lovers, but each relationship has ended because her lovers wanted more of her time than she felt comfortable spending away from her children. Currently she has no outside relationship.

Maria and Jorge are both nurses who work opposite shifts in a hospital. They are a married couple, and both are bisexual. Maria has a long-term sexual relationship with Rosa, a doctor on her shift, who comes home with Maria after work for romance and companionship while Jorge is working his shift at the hospital. Jorge has numerous affairs with other male nurses at night, while Maria and Rosa are at work.

Pros and Cons of the Primary/Secondary Model

This model is popular because it is the model most similar to traditional marriage and does not threaten the primacy of the couple. For most married or cohabiting couples, it is not such a stretch to have a few outside relationships as long as they know that the primary commitment is to the marriage. They can still be married, have children, live together, and be socially acceptable, keeping their outside relationships private from friends and family. One major benefit for many couples is that they feel secure that they won't be abandoned, because their spouse has agreed that outside relationships will be secondary. This model is simpler and easier to organize logistically than other forms of open relationships. If there is any conflict over time, loyalty or commitment, the spouse always gets priority.

However, a major drawback of this model is that outside relationships are not so simple or easy to predict or control. Having a sexual relationship with someone else often leads to becoming emotionally involved and falling in love, frequently causing a crisis in the primary relationship and sometimes triggering a divorce. Initiating a sexual relationship is opening a door to many possibilities, and often secondary relationships grow into something else which does not fit neatly into the confines of this model. Many people who are "secondary" lovers become angry at being subjugated to the couple, and demand equality or an end to the relationship. For this model to be successful, couples must be very convinced that their relationship is strong enough to weather these ups and downs. It is also wise to pick outside partners who are also partnered or are seeking a less committed relationship so they will be less likely to demand more time and attention than the primary relationship can comfortably allow.

It is a good idea for couples to talk over in advance what options will be considered in the event that a secondary relationship becomes something more serious than originally intended, as this is a very distinct possibility. One option is to end the secondary relationship and focus on strengthening the primary relationship before venturing into any new outside relationships. Another option is to try to "de-escalate" the situation by giving less time and attention to the secondary relationship in an effort to step back into a more casual relationship. A third option is to decide that this model isn't working and change to the Multiple Primary Partners model. Many couples who start with the Primary/Secondary model find that one or both people in the couple have become very emotionally attached to an outside relationship and decide eventually to shift to some form of the Multiple Primary Partners model, so that secondary relationships become equal to the primary couple relationship. Sometimes the partners are then called co-primaries.

Multiple Primary Partners Model

While there are many variations on this theme, the key factor is that all primary partner models include three or more people in a primary relationship in which all members are (or have the option of becoming) equal partners. Instead of a couple having priority and control in the relationship, all relationships are considered primary, or have the potential of becoming primary. Each partner has equal power to negotiate for what they want in the relationship, in terms of time, commitment, living situation, financial arrangements, sex, and other issues.

Some examples of variations on this model:

- *Polyfidelity Model—closed multi-adult families.* This is a "group marriage" model, essentially the same as being married — except you're married to more than one person. Such groups usually consist of three to six adults, with all partners living together and sharing finances, children, and household responsibilities. Depending on the sexual orientation of the members, all adults in the family may or may not be sexual partners. For instance, if all members are heterosexual, all the women have sexual relationships with all the men. If the women are bisexual, they may have sexual relationships with the women as well as the men. And so on. However, this is a closed system, and sex is only allowed between family members — no outside sexual relationships are allowed. Some families are open to taking on new partners, but only if all members of the family agree to accept the new person as a partner. The new person then moves into the household and becomes an equal member of the family.

  The polyfidelity model was made famous during the 1970s and 1980s by the Kerista commune in San Francisco, which had several households living in this model for many years. Other communal groups have implemented this model in various forms. Currently, the most common heterosexual form of this model is a triad of two women and one man, or two men and one woman. Many gay male triads also have lived happily together for decades. A few lesbian triads exist but are less common. And recently there have been a number of polyfidelitous families formed by two heterosexual couples who become a foursome and live together as a family.

For example:

Jane and Tom and Mary and Bill all live together as a polyfidelitous family. They have three children. They pool their incomes and make house payments, buy food, and provide for the children collectively, sharing child-rearing and household responsibilities. They are heterosexual, so each of the women has sexual relations with both men. Jane fell in love with Joaquin, an outside friend. After much consideration, all partners agreed that Joaquin could move into the household and join the family. He became an equal partner in the household and has sexual relationships with Jane and Mary.

Andre, Rachel and Nathan live together as a family; all three are bisexual. Rachel has sexual relationships with both Andre and Nathan. Andre and Nathan also have a sexual relationship. They have a "sleeping schedule" so that each relationship receives equal time, each spending two nights each week with each partner. They are hoping that another bisexual woman will join their family.

Pros and Cons of Polyfidelity

Polyfidelity can be a richly rewarding experience, creating an extended family and intentional community. Pooling resources is economical and ecological, and can reduce the stress of child rearing by spreading the work and the responsibility among several adults rather than just one or two parents. However, polyfidelity requires a very high level of compatibility and affinity between all partners. Living in a group requires excellent interpersonal skills, clear communication, assertiveness, co-operation, and flexibility in order to accommodate everyone's needs. Picking compatible partners and being accommodating are both key to successful polyfidelity. These issues will be explored in much greater detail in Chapter 12: "Living Styles for Polyamorous Families and Relationships."

- *Multiple Primary Partners — Open Model.* This model is very different from polyfidelity, in that all partners are given more autonomy and flexibility in developing any relationships they choose and defining those relationships on their own terms. In the Primary/Secondary model, the couple is the center of power, and in the polyfidelity model, the entire family group makes decisions together and all must agree. In the Multiple Primary Partners Open Model, the individual is the basic unit of the family and is empowered to make his or her own rules and decisions. Partners may choose to live together, or they may choose to live with one or more partners, or live alone if that better suits their needs. This model is open, in that each partner has the right to choose other lovers at any time without the approval of any other partner. Each relationship evolves independently of partners' other relationships, with rules and level of commitment to be negotiated by each individual. No one can veto a potential partner, or "pull rank" and insist on being the number one priority.

For example:

Jennifer and Andrea are a lesbian couple who live together. Andrea also has another primary partner, Julia, who does not live with them, but receives equal time and priority. Andrea spends one-half of each week with each woman.

Ricardo and Maria are a bisexual married couple; they spend Monday, Wednesday and Friday nights together. Tom also live with them, and has his own bedroom. Ricardo spends a few nights each week with Tom. Maria has two other lovers, Erica and Jessica.

Rita lives alone and she prefers having her own apartment. She has two committed, long-term relationships, with Bob and Jason, who also live alone. Bob and Jason each come to visit her at her apartment a few nights a week.

There is much more fluidity in the open-model approach, as relationships are allowed to evolve over time with very few rules to direct or restrict their direction or level of commitment. Many poly people experience this as a more organic approach to relationships, because each relationship can naturally rise to its own level without being molded by outside constraints. However, it is also much less predictable and may cause anxiety for people who like more structure and prefer a clear hierarchy.

Because all partners are considered equal, each partner can negotiate for what they want. However, all this "processing" requires time, effort, and excellent communication skills. And some people find the potential for conflicting loyalties to be too threatening. For instance, which partner will spend holidays or vacations with you? Will they both go, will they alternate each year, will you spend part of each holiday or vacation with each one? If one partner is going through a crisis, can they demand more of your time and commitment? If you are experiencing problems in one relationship or feel more drawn toward another partner during a given period of time, what behavior is appropriate? Weighing your own needs as well as the desires of each partner can be very stressful and confusing. Some people find this model requires too much thinking, problem-solving and creates too many confusing ethical and logistical dilemmas. Those who prefer a more rigid structure might do better with as the primary-secondary model or the polyfidelity model.

- *Multiple Non-Primary Relationships.* While the first two models stress commitment and primary relationships, some people prefer to remain essentially single but participate in more than one relationship. They are not looking for a committed relationship. For them, non-monogamy offers the intimacy, companionship, love, and sexual satisfaction of involvement in relationships, without the constraints of a primary relationship. This model generally works best for people who have a serious, all-consuming commitment to something other than relationships; people who are very busy with their work, their art, raising children alone, or political involvements. Usually they prefer relationships with people who, like themselves, want less commitment, or people who already have a primary relationship and are looking for a "secondary" relationship. People involved in this model usually don't make a lot of rules about their relationships, and retain a very high degree of personal freedom and autonomy. They usually live alone and make relationships a relatively low priority in their lives.

Some examples:

Juan is an artist who needs lots of time alone to paint. He has three lovers — Maria, Janice, and Keiko. He sees each of them regularly, usually making a date with each one every one to two weeks. Keiko and Janice are both married and see Juan when their husbands are at work or away on business. Maria is working on her Ph.D. dissertation, and has little time and energy for relationships. All three are too busy to seek a primary relationship with Juan.

Jessica is a single mother with three kids and a full time job. She has two long-term but casual sexual relationships with Jacob and Anthony. Jacob is a business executive who travels a lot for his job, so he is only free to see Jessica about once a week. Anthony is married to a bartender, and they have agreed to the Primary/Secondary model. As a result, he sees Jessica one evening a week when his wife is working.

For this model to be successful, it is crucial to choose partners who will be satisfied with a less committed relationship, and to communicate those intentions clearly to potential partners. However, conflict can arise when circumstances change and one person has more time or develops a desire for a primary relationship. For instance, when Maria finishes her dissertation, or when Jacob gets a promotion and no longer has to travel for his job, or a married lover gets divorced — they may suddenly demand more time and commitment or even demand a monogamous relationship. Such a change often proves fatal to the existing relationships. However, sometimes people see such a challenge as an opportunity for growth and are able to change their relationship to accommodate everyone's needs.

A Few Words on Poly Models

There are many different types of open relationships. Some models will fit your needs much better than others. To identify your preferred model, ask yourself some tough questions: How much security do you need to feel safe in a relationship? Do you need to feel that you're

"Number One," or can you share that priority with other lovers? How much privacy and personal freedom do you need to feel comfortable? Have you been happiest living alone, living with one person, or with a group? What has pushed your buttons in past relationships? How much time and energy do you have to devote to relationships? What are your expectations of love relationships?

Last, but certainly not least, it is crucial to pick partners who want the same type of relationship and are comfortable with your chosen model. Excellent interpersonal and communications skills go a long way towards achieving these goals, along with a willingness to negotiate to satisfy everyone's needs.

Now you have an idea of the three major types of open relationships, and the benefits and drawbacks of each model. The next step is to learn the skills that will maximize your chances of developing satisfying and successful open relationships. Part Two covers the four steps towards developing the basic skill set needed for this type of relationship.

·

PART TWO
Building Your Polyamory Skill Set

3
Four Steps to Poly Relating

Step 1: Examine Your Motives.

Most people have a complex mix of motives for entering relationships, and often we are not even sure ourselves what combination of variables is driving us to enter a particular relationship or type of relationship. Polyamorous people may feel even less certain about such issues, as we may have a different set of motives for getting involved in a primary couple relationship or marriage than for seeking other partners.

We can save ourselves and our partners a lot of suffering by taking a long, hard look at what is motivating us to choose a polyamorous love life in the first place. Often we are defensive about these issues and reluctant to address them seriously, partly because so often these questions are thrown in our faces in a judgmental manner by monogamous people who disapprove of our relationships. When they ask us, "Why do you need to have more than one partner?" the implication is that there is something wrong with us because we "just can't be satisfied" with one, monogamous relationship. However, if we can get over our knee-jerk reactions and understand what we hope to receive and experience through having more than one partner or relationship, we are much more likely to be successful in actually creating happy and healthy relationships.

Whether monogamous or polyamorous, most people are drawn to their relationship orientation by a mixture of healthy and unhealthy motives.

For example, monogamous people may be motivated toward monogamy as a way of life for any or all of the following reasons:

- They believe that monogamy will lead to security and stability, and that exclusivity will enhance their experience of intimacy and love.

- They hope that monogamy will create a stable family life for their children.

- They want to demonstrate their commitment to their partner through sexual fidelity.

- They want to please their parents and be accepted by their peers.

- They do not want to confront the possibility that their partner could be sexually or romantically interested in someone else, and do not want to deal with their own jealousy or a jealous partner.

- Monogamy seems simpler and they don't want to commit the time and energy required for managing multiple relationships.

- Monogamy is the only acceptable path in their religion or culture.

- They are willing to sacrifice sexual variety to make their partner feel special and loved.

Many of those motives are healthy and demonstrate maturity, strength of character, and commitment to their partner, but others indicate insecurities, dependence, and unquestioning conformity.

By the same token, polyamorous people may be motivated to seek multiple partners for any or all of the following reasons:

- We are adventurous and willing to chart our own relationship path despite religious and societal disapproval.

- We want more sex and more sexual variety and feel sexually unsatisfied with just one partner.

- We have a need for more attention, stimulation, and companionship than the average person.

- We feel a need to validate our desirability by being wanted by new partners.

- We use sex and relationships to medicate depression, anxiety, boredom, or loneliness.

- We value freedom and don't want to be constrained by one relationship.

- We are afraid to commit fully to one person.

- We are afraid of intimacy and fully disclosing who we are to our partners.

- We use multiple relationships to try to make up for some real or perceived lack of love in our childhood or our past.

- We don't feel secure in any one relationship and are "hedging our bets" by having multiple partners so we won't be alone if one partner leaves us.

Many of these motives indicate independence, courage, willingness to try something that is non-traditional, challenging ourselves to personal growth, risking the loss of social acceptance in order to follow our own path. However, some polyamorous people are driven by compulsive behaviors, self-indulgence, fear of intimacy or commitment, and immaturity.

While each person has a unique combination of variables which drive us towards a particular relationship orientation, no one is perfect. It's a rare person that can honestly say that their motives are entirely "clean." We can benefit from admitting that some of our motives come from our own wounding in past adult relationships and/or our childhood traumas and insecurities, as this gives us greater understanding of our complex needs and allows us to make more conscious choices about our relationships. Owning our motives and taking responsibility for our needs also allows us to be honest with our partners about what we are seeking and enables them to make an informed decision about whether to choose a relationship with us.

Exercise for discerning your motives. **Taking a few minutes to do the following exercise may give you useful information about your relationship motives and goals:**

Sit quietly for a few minutes and think about your life experience with monogamous relationships, your memories of your parents' relationship(s), your own monogamous relationships in the past, and other monogamous relationships

of friends or family you have witnessed. Write down on a piece of paper all the things you like about monogamy in general and those relationships specifically, and all the reasons you could possibly imagine being monogamous. Then write down all the things you dislike about monogamy and monogamous relationships you have been in or have seen in others. Then, try to complete the sentence "I would be happy to be monogamous if..." by trying to imagine if there are some conditions which would be likely to make you happy in a monogamous relationship. Then try to complete the sentence, "The things I fear and dread the most about monogamy are..." Another sentence that can be revealing is "The things I hated most about being in an monogamous relationship were..."

Then, think for a few minutes about open relationships, and everything you know about them or have experienced personally. Write down all the things you find attractive about polyamory and the good things you have experienced in open relationships or have seen in other people's polyamorous relationships. Then, try to complete the sentence, "I want to be polyamorous because..." Be as honest as you can about your needs, desires, and motives, and read your list over carefully to see if you have learned anything new about your orientation toward open relationships. Then complete the sentence "The things I hope to experience and receive in polyamorous relationships are..."

If you see some unhealthy motives on your list, be compassionate with yourself and understand that we all have areas where we have room for personal growth. These are areas you may want to work on either on your own or by taking classes, reading books, or seeking a support group or therapist.

Step 2: Know which model is right for you, and make appropriate agreements with your partner(s).

Most people decide to try a polyamorous lifestyle or accidentally stumble into an open relationship without thinking carefully about what type of relationship they actually want and what agreements they need to feel safe and loved. While it is ideal to try to figure out what model of open relationship will work best for you before you enter into it, most people do not realize until they are in the middle of it that they need some boundaries and rules. And some people can only find out what works for them by trying one model and realizing that it makes them miserable, and then trying a different model.

As we discussed in Chapter 2, there are three basic models of open relationships. To refresh your memory, they are:

- The primary/secondary model: In this model, couple establishes a committed primary relationship, and agrees to have only secondary relationships outside their relationship.

- The multiple primary partners model, with two variations:

    The closed model, called polyfidelity, which is a group marriage with multiple partners who are sexually exclusive within that group, and

    The open model, where any and all relationships have the potential of becoming primary.

- The multiple non-primary partners model: All relationships are casual or secondary, and there is no primary relationship.

You will create intense suffering for all concerned if you want one model and your partner or partners desire another model, as these models are mutually exclusive. Some people are able to successfully transition from one model to another when they discover that the model they are in does not work for them, but often this is quite painful and not all partners will accept the change.

How can you know which model is right for you? Start by asking yourself which past relationship made you the happiest. What was it about that relationship that seemed so healthy and satisfying for you?

You may discover additional important information by asking yourself, what is the past relationship in which you were least happy? As you think about that, pay attention to your feelings about this past relationship as you identify the qualities in that relationship that made you miserable. In going over these past relationships and what made them satisfying or unhappy for you, you will begin to see what characteristics you want (and don't want) in relationships. This will enable you to decide which model is most likely to work you, and help you make relationship agreements you will be able to keep.

You can use this checklist to help you see patterns and clarify your preferred model.

For instance, you are likely to be happiest with the primary/secondary model if you were happiest in a relationship where:

- You were in a primary partnership with one person and no other primary relationships existed,
- You had a regular routine and schedule that you could count on over time,
- You had veto power over your partner's choice of other partners,
- You spent most of your free time with a primary partner, including weekends, holidays, and vacations,
- You and your partner expected a high level of accountability to each other (for instance, you always told each other where you were going, checked in frequently, accounted for your time, money, and activities),
- You or your partner became uncomfortable or insecure if an outside partner began to demand too much time and attention, and/or
- The relationship was very committed and stable.

Conversely, you are likely to be most satisfied with the closed multiple primary partners/polyfidelity model if you were happiest in a past relationship where

- You lived with more than one partner and enjoyed the companionship of more than one domestic partner,
- You spent most of your time together with multiple partners on a daily, weekly, and monthly basis,
- You were very flexible and accommodating, and willing to compromise with your partners,
- You appreciated your partners checking in frequently, being accountable to each other for their time and activities,
- The relationship was very committed and stable,

- You didn't experience a lot of jealousy and insecurity when your other partners were connecting,
- There was a lot of structure and routine,
- You had veto power over your partner's choice of other partners, and
- You were comfortable with less privacy and personal freedom.

You are most likely to do best with the multiple primary partners "open model" if you were happiest in a past relationship where:

- You were comfortable with a lot of fluidity and change in relationships, with relationships sometimes evolving from secondary to primary,
- You were able to successfully juggle more than one primary relationship,
- You demonstrated excellent time management skills,
- You were able to manage your own insecurities and jealousy reasonably well,
- You enjoyed or could tolerate re-negotiating boundaries and agreements from time to time,
- You thrived on having more freedom and privacy, and were able to tolerate your partners having a similar degree of autonomy and privacy,
- You were comfortable with less structure and routine in that relationship, and
- You did not have veto power over your partner's choice of other partners.

You are most likely to enjoy the multiple non-primary partners model if you were most satisfied with a past relationship where:

- Your needs for intimacy and companionship were well met by one or more casual or secondary relationships,
- You had complete control over your schedule, your time, and your activities,

- You lived alone or with roommates or family members who were not lovers,

- You spent a relatively small amount of your time with partners,

- You were focused on another commitment such as work or school which demanded the bulk of your time and attention.

While this checklist is of course not exhaustive and certainly not foolproof, it can help you identify the characteristics most important to you in the different models of open relationships. It is imperative that you be brutally honest with yourself and your partners about what you need in a relationship model, and make agreements based on your actual needs. It is tempting to base our agreements on what we wish were true for us or who we would like to be, rather than on the reality of what kind of relationship will actually work for us. This is especially true when a partner or potential partner is more oriented toward a different relationship model and is pressuring you to move towards their model. This situation usually creates unhappiness for all concerned and is unlikely to be sustainable over time.

Step 3: Pick compatible partners

This advice may seem painfully obvious, but is necessary to reiterate. The single most common mistake made by polyamorous people is to get into relationships with people who are not polyamorous. This mistake is certain to doom any relationship, because people who want open relationships are not compatible with partners who have a monogamous orientation. Just as dangerous are partners that quietly or reluctantly go along with an open relationship, while harboring the illusion that their partner will eventually choose monogamy to be with them. Most monogamists cannot be converted, nor will polyamorists become monogamous. The odds are extremely slim that a relationship can survive between people who have relationship orientations that are mutually exclusive. When you are smitten with a wonderful person, it is tempting to believe that love can conquer all, but irreconcilable differences will rapidly become fatal to the relationship when the infatuation wears off and all the projection and fantasy starts to give way to reality.

By the same token, it can be just as disastrous to choose partners who do not want the same type of open relationship that you do. If you have a primary partner and are seeking secondary partners, don't get involved with someone who is single and looking for a primary. They will experience a scarcity of time and attention and become needy and demanding, and you will feel guilty and overwhelmed by competing demands. While it may seem obvious that this is a bad idea, it is the second most common mistake in open relationships: starting a secondary relationship with someone who wants a primary relationship. Sometimes this is an honest mistake that cannot be avoided, as people often get involved in casual or secondary relationships which gradually become a lot more serious. It is not always possible to predict how you are going to feel about someone at the beginning of what seems like a brief fling or a very part-time relationship. One or both parties may discover a much deeper connection growing between them, and then they may have to reassess and may terminate their relationship. Sometimes it is possible to negotiate with their primary partner(s) to expand the relationship to a primary relationship if everyone consents, but often this is not possible.

And in any kind of intimate relationship, whether open or monogamous, a good rule of thumb is to avoid getting involved with anyone who has a lot more emotional problems than you do. While this suggestion may seem as obvious as the previous advice about picking compatible partners, it is the third most common mistake in open relationships. Some poly people have a habit of picking partners who have emotional wounding or are mentally unstable and will create drama and crises everywhere they go. While that can be daunting enough in a monogamous relationship, in an open relationship it is likely to condemn the relationship. If you have a monogamous partner who has meltdowns, throws tantrums, or makes unreasonable demands, the extra processing and chaos only affect you and your partner. In an open relationship, every relationship in the intimate circle is disrupted by the problems created by one unstable person. The drama with one partner causes a domino effect on your other partner(s), your partner's other partner(s), etc.

For example:

Jorge was married to Joan, and they had a very stable primary relationship. However, he got involved in a very tempestuous outside relationship with Donna, who often

became jealous when Jorge was spending time with his wife. She would call their house repeatedly throughout the day and night, crying and demanding that Jorge come to her house immediately to comfort her. The first few times, Joan urged him to go to Donna and spend a little time with her to help her feel more secure. Joan hoped that this would help Donna manage her feelings when Jorge was spending time at home. However, Donna's demands escalated and soon she was driving over to their house and banging on the door screaming, "I know you're in there with her! Come out here right now!" By this time Joan was not feeling so generous towards Donna and insisted that Jorge send her home with a promise to talk with her in the morning. These incidents disrupted Joan and Jorge's relationship, causing a crisis which required a lot of time for processing and, eventually, couples counseling. This in turn affected Joan's outside relationship with Jennifer, because her problems with Jorge were taking so much time and energy that she was neglecting her other relationship. Jennifer was so unhappy with Joan being distracted and upset with Jorge over the situation with Donna, that she eventually got fed up and left the relationship.

Many people in open relationships make this mistake once, and have such a terrible experience that they learn to carefully assess potential partners for their stability, emotional health, interpersonal skills, and track record in relationships.

For example:

Jamal is a gay man in a committed, long-term relationship with Jason. He explains, "I had a crazy love affair with a drama queen for a year, and nearly lost my husband and my sanity before I finally came to my senses." He knew from the start that Harris, the new boyfriend, liked drugs and partying, but thought that because it was a secondary relationship that they could "just have a good time together and keep it casual." And because his primary relationship was so stable and happy, he thought he could tolerate a little instability in his outside relationship without any ill effects. However, it proved impossible to keep it from spilling over into his life as Harris spiraled into a methamphetamine addiction. He started stealing money from Jamal, showing up at his workplace on drugs, and calling Jason in the middle of the night spouting paranoia and threats. This caused Jason to pack his bags and leave, staying with his other partner for a month until Jamal was able to extricate himself from this destructive relationship, get a restraining order to keep Harris away from his home and workplace, and plead with Jason to give him another chance to prove he could make their primary relationship work.

No partner, primary or otherwise, is perfect. Sometimes it is impossible to tell at the beginning of a new relationship if this new partner will be wonderful and interesting, or way too high-maintenance to manage. People are on their best behavior on those crucial first few dates, and we are under the influence of lust and infatuation, so mistakes are made. Being in an open relationship requires being willing to go through some trial and error as each person learns how to pick appropriate partners and figures out what kind of relationships, and how many, they can handle.

Step Four: Build on a Firm Foundation

When you build a house, it doesn't matter how beautiful the house is if the foundation is crumbling or not strong enough to hold the weight of the house. For much the same reason, you cannot build an open relationship if there are some serious problems in your current relationship. Initiating an open relationship will be certain to create conflict and problems in your primary relationship, and that relationship needs to be healthy, strong, and stable enough to tolerate the stress that is sure to be generated. Think carefully about whether your relationship has any glaring problems that need to be addressed and resolved before you consider opening up your relationship to other partners. This may seem extremely self-evident. However, I see many couples who have ignored serious problems in their relationship and jumped into a polyamorous relationship. Those same problems have followed them into the new relationships they have added, as well as inflamed the conflicts in their own relationship.

Even worse, many couples mistakenly believe that polyamory will fix existing problems in their relationship, only to find that it has made them worse. While having outside relationships can enhance your relationship and ameliorate certain problems, looking to polyamory to solve your problems as a couple is fraught with peril.

Why? As discussed in Chapter One, most polyamorous people are looking for "Different" or "More." In other words, they want outside relationships because they are happy with what they receive in their current relationship, but also want something different that is not available, such as a different kind of sex, or a different gender partner, or a partner who is more affectionate or more emotional. Or they love their current relationship but do not receive enough of something, such as sex, time, attention, romance, intimacy, and want to "supplement" that by having another partner. For a couple that has a relationship that is pretty healthy and happy, these discrepancies can be solved through an open relationship, as each person can meet their needs for "more" or "different" through outside relationships. However, if there are serious problems and incompatibilities in a relationship, they will only be worsened by polyamory: partners gradually start to meet most or all of their needs for satisfaction and emotional connection outside their primary relationship, and that relationship becomes distant and strained, and eventually dies. So it is important to think carefully about what needs you are trying to meet in outside relationships and how that may affect your primary relationship.

Most important, take care of your own relationship first. Work with your partner to improve your communication skills, and consider seeking couples counseling and/or individual counseling to enhance your relationship and address outstanding problems. Take the time and effort necessary to deepen your level of intimacy with your partner and increase your trust. Now that you understand the different models and the basic steps to creating healthy open relationships, the next two chapters will cover communication skills specifically designed for polyamorous relationships, as well as the most common communication problems you are likely to encounter in open relationships.

4 Poly Communication Skills 1.0

While excellent communication skills are a prerequisite for any healthy, happy relationship, they are even more important in polyamorous relationships. This is because monogamous couples often can get by, at least for awhile, on assumptions and expectations that are based on the model of the traditional heterosexual marriage. People in open relationships are in a whole different ball game. We cannot count on any of our partners having the same rules in mind unless we clearly voice our needs and boundaries and make explicit relationship agreements. As a result, it is very important for people in open relationships to learn to communicate clearly and to err on the side of more communication rather than less. Communication skills take time and effort to learn and practice, but are well worth the effort, as they pay huge dividends in sustaining healthy relationships.

Don't look for complex formulas for polyamorous communication. In fact, it is most important to tend to the basics and keep communication as simple as possible. Any communication techniques must be simple enough for you and your partners to utilize them when there is a conflict, emotions are high, and no one is thinking clearly. When one or more people are feeling angry, hurt, jealous, or just plain irrational due to intense feelings, any complicated communication technique is likely to go out the window. So for any communication skill to be useful, it has to be simple and easy enough to remember and use when you or your partner(s) are at your worst.

In the absence of clear communication, one or more partner(s) may feel unheard, and may resort to strategies to undermine new relationships — such as the individual who says "yes" to their primary partner's request to start an outside relationship, but then vetoes the new partner for some rather dubious or contrived reason, makes rules that are so unreasonable that the potential lover loses interest, or deliberately plans social events that keep their partner from successfully making dates with the new person. Polyamorous people can save themselves and their partner(s) a lot of anguish by paying close attention to and immediately addressing their words, non-verbal communication, and behaviors.

In my experience these are the most important things to remember in communicating with your partner(s) and resolving polyamorous dilemmas.

- *Listen carefully!* Pay close attention to your partner's words, non-verbal communications, and actions. This may sound like stating the ridiculously obvious, but I see couples every day for counseling who have gotten into a world of trouble because they have not been listening to each other. This is often most true in long-term relationships, as there is an unfortunate tendency to think we know our partners so well that we no longer have to listen to them.

- *Pay attention to more than words.* Another common communication pitfall is to hear the words but ignore the body language, tone of voice, and other non-verbal communication that often speak much louder than words if we only pay attention. This is especially true in open relationships where one partner may feel pressured to go along with something their partner requests — for instance, wanting to spend the weekend with another partner or wanting to have unprotected sex with another partner — even if they have strong negative feelings about granting permission. In these situations, a partner may say yes but all their non-verbal signals are saying no, and it is imperative to "hear" that non-verbal communication and address your partner's misgivings directly and lovingly to attempt some resolution of the issue. Usually, this involves either suggesting a compromise or agreeing to postpone this request until your partner can verbalize their feelings and problem-solve to feel safer. Many couples have created major drama and pain by ignoring all the non-verbal signs that something was not really okay even though the partner ostensibly agreed to it.

- ***Know what you want and need, and communicate it directly to your partner(s).*** For many couples and individuals who are exploring open relationships, knowing what we want and need can be very challenging, as this may all be new and unfamiliar. Often "trial and error" is the only path to discovering what works and doesn't work, and what boundaries and rules we may need to safely evolve into a polyamorous lifestyle.

For instance, you may think it is fine to consent to your partner's request to have a date with a new person and pursue sex and romance with this new lover. However, when said partner actually does so, you may become distraught. It may take awhile to pinpoint what is distressing about this situation and what you need from your partner to feel safe and loved. It may be that this particular person triggers jealousy for some reason, or this may be a bad time for you because of other stresses in life, or you may be going through a lot of conflict in your relationship already and the relationship can't handle the additional stress of this new partner at this moment. As soon as you are able to discern what you want, directly but gently express these feelings to your partner, acknowledging that you did actually consent to this, but that you have found that you need a change in the agreement since this is creating more pain than you can tolerate right now. Make your best guess about what your bottom line is and stick to that, while trying to stretch yourself and consent to something that may be very uncomfortable but not intolerable. Be compassionate with yourself and your partner(s) as you go through this process; since it is so stressful and unpredictable, each change will create some inconvenience and distress for everyone.

Because these guidelines often are a moving target, this can cause resentments and disappointment for everyone along the way. Often this feels like "going backwards" to the partner with an outside relationship, because they usually ask for more time and greater freedom to pursue the outside relationship, while their primary partner may be asking them to give up some of the things that have been agreed on as they can't tolerate as much as they originally thought.

For example:

Jose agreed to allow his primary partner, Peter, to have sex with his ex-boyfriend, Gregg, who was going to be in town for a week on business. Jose agreed that Peter and Gregg could spend three nights together since Gregg would only be in town for such a short time. However, after the first night, Jose felt terrible and asked Peter to come home and spend the next night with him. Peter was angry because Jose had "broken his agreement," but consented and they were able to make a new agreement that Peter could have two nights with Gregg instead of three.

Joan agreed that her husband Bill could have sex with and spend the night with his outside partner Robin. Bill had two dates with her but Joan experienced intense jealousy and insomnia both nights. She asked him to continue dating Robin and having sex with her but not to spend the night, until she could get her anxieties under control. He was unhappy with this change and Robin felt hurt and betrayed, but Bill agreed. After a few more dates, Joan felt comfortable enough to give her consent to him spending the night with Robin again.

The two keys to successfully communicating your needs to your partner(s) are: being willing to admit that you have guessed wrong about what you can handle, and telling the truth about your needs even though you know your partner will not be happy with what you are asking for. We all have a tendency to tell our partners what we think they want to hear, and to go along with things that will not work for us. It is almost always better to be honest about your feelings and ask as clearly as possible for what you need, and be willing to compromise if you can to make it work better for everyone.

Here's a helpful exercise when you're faced with a difficult decision on polyamorous boundaries. Ask yourself these three questions:

- **What would be absolutely ideal for me in this situation?**

- **What would be difficult and painful but likely to be manageable with some work on my part and support from my partner(s) and others?**

- **What would make me really unhappy in this situation right now?**

Don't hesitate to say no to any relationship guideline or boundary that fails the last question. You may feel a lot of pressure from your partner or your partner's other partner(s) to make more compromises or go along with something they really want, and many people in open relationships have made the mistake of "being a good sport," "being flexible," "challenging yourself," or "doing this for your own personal growth." However, if you push yourself to accept something that makes you feel fundamentally unsafe or makes you feel mistreated or unloved, you will regret making that agreement and it will cause more harm than good in your relationship.

If you are uncertain about whether a particular request or guideline is tolerable for you, negotiate a default or fall-back plan before implementing this new practice, so that you have a way to re-open the discussion if it proves too difficult. For instance, you could agree to try something for a month and then re-evaluate to see whether to continue. Or you can agree to accept a range of behaviors with the caveat that if any one of these become too painful or create too much stress in your relationship, you can opt to veto one of the practices for a period of time. Again, clear and honest communication is imperative, to express what is okay and what has turned out to be too difficult.

Tell the truth!

The third crucial step in communication in poly relationships is to tell your partner(s) the truth about yourself, your feelings, and your outside sexual and romantic relationships. The appropriate amount of disclosure is very important, so that your partners know what is going on in your life and how it will affect them. However, there is no formula for how much disclosure is best, as each person and each relationship has a different constellation of needs for privacy and for information. It is a very delicate and complicated process to create the right balance between allowing each person and each individual relationship to have some privacy while providing all partners with enough information to feel safe, respected, and up to date. Later in this chapter you will learn about how to assess your own and your partners' needs around disclosure, as it is a very common sore spot in poly relationships.

However, the most important rule of thumb is: don't lie! If a partner asks you a question you don't want to answer, or requests information you would rather keep private, lying is the worst possible response. While it may cause conflict and pain, it is always better to say, "I really don't want to talk about that," or "My partner would prefer I don't share that information with you," or "I understand your desire to know more, but I don't feel comfortable disclosing that." Another approach is to ask your partner why they want this information, and what they hope to achieve by knowing more about this aspect of your life or other relationships. Often, this question will lead to a more fruitful discussion about your partner's needs and their motivation for asking for more disclosure, and usually it will become clear that there is another way to reassure them or reduce their anxieties without sharing information that you would prefer to keep private.

If you are caught off-guard by a partner's questioning and accidentally react by saying things that aren't true, don't panic. This is very common in poly situations and most people have done it at one time or another when they felt confused or defensive and just didn't know how to handle a partner's request for more disclosure than they felt willing to give. In open relationships there is a very strong temptation to lie about some parts of outside relationships, because we have never had any training in how to talk with a partner about another concurrent relationship: doing so seems so counter-intuitive that our default programming is to lie.

As soon as you realize you have told your partner some half-truths or untruths, or as soon afterward as you can muster the courage, take a few deep breaths and acknowledge that you have made a mistake and that you would like to clear up the misunderstanding. This takes a lot of integrity and maturity, but it is well worth the stress of dealing with your partner feeling hurt and suspicious because of your behavior. You will cause much more damage by letting a lie stand (and pay a much higher price for it later) than by just correcting the mistake as soon as possible.

One way to make this process easier is to practice this skill in a non-charged situation, when there is no outside relationship going on. Some couples practice by telling each other about random people they find attractive, such as strangers on the street or movie stars, just to get in the habit of talking about this subject, so it will be easier when there is a real situation to address. Others practice by talking about past relationships they had prior to the current primary relationship, because it may feel easier to talk about and to hear about since the relationship is over and in the past.

Metacommunicate!

Philosopher Gregory Bateson invented the term "metacommunicate" in the 1970s to describe the idea of "communicating about communication." This is a very useful concept for all relationships, but especially for open relationships. The idea is to communicate the goal of your communication to your partner before you start talking about the subject itself. This allows your partner to get an idea of what you are trying to achieve with this discussion and can stay on track with reaching that goal. It is important to recognize that people often have different goals when they communicate, and this can cause a great deal of conflict and miscommunication. The comedian Lily Tomlin once said that humans invented communication and language because we have a primal need to complain, and that language facilitated whining. Another comedian, Robin Williams, contends that language was invented by men to woo women. He says that men figured out that it was a lot easier to get laid if they talked to a woman. While there is certainly merit to both of these philosophies, in my experience, people communicate for five different reasons. Usually an individual is trying to achieve one of these five goals through a particular communication:

1) To make a connection with your partner, to create closeness and intimacy:

"I'm happy to see you."

"How was your day today?"

"I missed you and I wanted to talk to you."

"I was just thinking about that romantic vacation we took five years ago to Mexico and how much fun we had."

2) To tell a story or give your partner information:

"My mom called and she is going to come by tomorrow."

"I ran into my friend Jan and she's pregnant!"

"This funny thing happened at work today and I think you will get a kick out of it."

"A package came for you today."

3) To ask for support or comfort:

"I had a migraine today and it was rough getting through the day at work."

"I feel sad because you snapped at me this morning and I need reassurance that you aren't mad at me."

"I'm really tired and I would love a back rub."

4) To solve a problem together:

"We got a bill from the IRS today and I need your help to figure out if we did something wrong on our taxes."

"We have been arguing lately and I don't know what to do about it."

"Your mother wants us to come for Thanksgiving and I don't really want to go."

5. To make a decision together:

"What color should we paint the kitchen?"

"I'd like your help in deciding whether I should take this part-time job or hold out for a full-time job."

"I'd like to take a vacation this year, and we need to decide if we can afford it or not."

It can be extremely useful to think about what the purpose of your communication is before starting the conversation with your partner, and communicate that goal to your partner. For instance, if you let your partner know that you are just trying to relate a story or talking because you want to connect, they are much more likely to cooperate with that goal and not derail you by trying to solve a problem or make a decision, and you are both likely to be more satisfied with the conversation.

Because we are so influenced by our gender training and socialization, men and women often have different goals for communication. Women, who are strongly socialized to value relationships and connection, are more likely to communicate to achieve the first three goals: create intimacy or feel connected, tell a story, or ask for support or comfort. Men, trained to be analyze, to compete, and to "fix things," are more likely to see most communication as an attempt to solve problems or come to a decision. It is dangerous to make gross generalizations based on gender, as of course not all women and all men communicate in these stereotypical ways. However, a significant percentage of women do tend to be focused on communication goals 1, 2, and 3 as described above, and men tend to focus on 4 and 5. Goals 1, 2, and 3 can be viewed as more relational, while 4 and 5 can be seen as more technical or practical.

Because of their very different ways of approaching communication, men and women in heterosexual relationships often experience communication breakdowns. For instance, the woman in a couple may be talking about an unpleasant interaction with her boss at work that day, as a way of asking for nurturing and support from her partner. Instead, he interprets it as a problem to be solved, and makes numerous suggestions on how she could have handled the situation with her boss differently in order to create a more positive outcome. She feels invalidated, criticized, and defensive, and he is baffled and hurt because his sensible advice and attempts to help are being rejected. Conversely, a man may talk about feeling dissatisfied with his job as a way of getting input from his partner about whether to stay at this job or look for another job. He wants help in weighing the various factors in order to make a decision, but she thinks he just wants to vent and get support, so she praises him for his hard work and skills and tells him how much she loves him, and asks him to share his feelings about his work. He is frustrated because she is derailing him from his focus on decision-making. She feels hurt because he doesn't appreciate her support.

For many heterosexual couples, this is the quintessential communication problem: communicating to meet one goal, and your partner responding with a different goal in mind, and neither goal is achieved. For same-sex couples, this dynamic often still exists but is usually not as pronounced, as both partners have been socialized to communicate in similar ways.

To minimize these communication problems, it can really help to metacommunicate, to tell your partner what the goal of the communication is before you start talking about something. This way, your partner knows what to listen for and how best to respond in order to meet your stated goal. I worked with one couple who had a recurring argument because when the wife was talking about something, the husband would interrupt her and ask, "Should I be listening to this, or are you just talking?" This infuriated the wife and made her feel disregarded and ignored. However, his actual intention was to find out if he should be listening for the facts and details of what she was saying, because she would expect him to help her solve a problem or make a decision, or whether he should be listening to the feelings and the flow of the conversation because she was just trying to connect, tell a story, or get support. He was really trying to metacommunicate, to ask her about the goal of the communication she was delivering.

I often suggest that couples try the following exercise. Think of something you want to communicate to your partner, and think about what you hope to achieve by delivering that communication. Tell your partner as clearly as you can what is the goal of your communication, and have them confirm that they understand the goal. Then start talking with your partner just as you normally would about this subject. You will probably be surprised at how much more your partner will "get" what you are trying to say, and they are much more likely to respond in the way you had wished.

For example:

A bisexual couple, Benjamin and Molly, in which Benjamin is making an effort to metacommunicate. Benjamin starts by saying, "I'd like to talk with you about something that is going on with my other partner, Jim. I would like your help in making a decision, but I also want to express my feelings about something and be heard and supported. And I want to hear your feelings and address any concerns you have before making this decision." Molly responds that she will try to listen carefully and give her support, and will give her honest feedback and any problems she might see in this situation, so they can come to a decision together.

Benjamin continues, "Jim has made a request that he would like us to stop using condoms and become fluid-bonded. It would mean a lot to him and allow him to feel more intimate, since he knows that we are fluid-bonded and he feels like he is being distrusted and seen as a vector of disease, and that makes him feel very hurt. He does not have any other partners now and has recently been re-tested and is negative for all STDs, including HIV. I have mixed feelings about taking this step, as it would be the first time we have agreed to having unprotected sex with anyone outside of our marriage. However, I feel that since Jim and I have been lovers for three years now and have a committed relationship, it seems reasonable to make this request."

Molly responds, "I can understand why both you and Jim would want this, and can see how he feels he isn't being treated fairly. I understand your mixed feelings, as I also am ambivalent about whether I might feel hurt by not being the only one you are fluid-bonded with. I also have some anxieties about being at risk for HIV or STDs, as I don't know Jim's history or his current sexual practices."

Benjamin says, "I don't believe it would put you or me at risk, as I completely trust Jim to tell me if he sleeps with any new partners and we can reconsider this if and when he gets involved with someone else."

Molly responds, "I do trust him, as he has always treated our relationship respectfully and has always been honest with both of us. But I'm not sure I'm ready to make this decision. As a compromise, since you would like to make a decision now, could we try going forward with this for a month and see how we both feel about it?"

Benjamin suggests, "Let's wait on making a decision, and talk about it again in a couple of weeks after we both have had time to think it through and express any feelings or concerns we have."

Because Benjamin started the conversation by stating clearly the goals of the communication, it is much easier for he and Molly to hear each other, validate each other's feelings, and work towards a mutually satisfying solution.

5 Common Communication Breakdowns in Open Relationships

While communication can be very challenging in any kind of intimate relationship, two specific communication issues are specific to open relationships: first, problems regarding disclosure about other relationships; and second, lack of clarity about the goal of your communication.

Disclosure: What Do You Really Want Or Need to Know?

When I was a nurse working in an Intensive Care Unit, it became clear to me that there were two types of patients. One type wanted to learn everything about their illness and know everything about the medications and treatments they were receiving, and wanted advance notice of any procedure or anything that was going to happen so they could be prepared for it. Having more information made them feel empowered, like they were a participant in their health care, and feel safer that there would be no surprises. Having less information made them feel vulnerable, helpless, and out of control.

The other type of patient wanted very little information about their illness. The more they learned about their condition and treatment, the more they obsessed about every possible symptom and complication, and they became more anxious about illness and even death. They would be haunted by terrifying images of surgeries, medical procedures, complications, and permanent disability and death that could possibly result from their illness or from the treatments they were receiving.

These two groups had very different needs for disclosure about their condition and treatments, because of their opposite coping strategies for handling potentially distressing information.

Similarly, there are two types of polyamorous people when it comes to how much disclosure they want about their partner's other relationships: those that want as much information as possible and want to know everything about their partner's other lovers and what is going on in those relationships, and those who want very little information about outside relationships. This seems to be linked to different personality styles.

For those who want to know everything, knowledge is power and having more information makes them feel safer. The more they know about their partner's other relationships, the more secure they feel. This knowledge reassures them that they know where they stand with their partner, and how their relationship fits into the bigger picture. They feel less anxious about possible surprises or reversals of fortune if they are keeping close track of what is going on with other relationships that may affect them.

Sometimes, however, their thirst for information is overzealous, and they want to know so much about the other partners that it becomes intrusive and their partner feels harassed and defensive. Often they ask a thousand questions and their partner in exasperation will say, "Why do you need to know all this?" This is an excellent question and you can save yourself and your partners a lot of grief by thinking carefully about what you really need to know and why. What are the crucial pieces of information you need about your partner's other relationships and how will having this information help you? Most often, if someone asks a lot of questions and demands a lot of detailed information, what they really want to know is this: "Is this other relationship a threat to the stability or survival of my relationship? Am I in danger of being displaced or replaced by this other person?" Usually, if you can answer that question honestly and reassure your partner that they are safe and loved, their need for constant updates is likely to subside. If you can respond to those very primal fears of abandonment and scarcity, all the other questions become irrelevant.

Some partners, on the other hand, prefer to have very little information about their partner's other relationships, and don't ask many questions. For this group, the more they know about a partner's outside relationships, the more anxious they become. Having more information only gives them more distressing facts to focus on, and encourages them to obsess about uncomfortable images of their partner with another lover. Hearing more about the relationship only convinces them that it must be really serious if you are talking about it so much, and each time you bring it up they fear you are going to announce that you are breaking up with them to be with this other partner. Their way of handling their partner having other partners is to compartmentalize the other relationships and focus on their own relationship and their own life activities, not giving a lot of attention or thought to what their partner may be doing with anyone else.

It is a mistake to try to force this type of partner to talk more about their partner's other relationships or about their feelings about them, as this will only create problems where none exist.

Many couples find that one person in the couple is in the first camp of wanting a high level of disclosure, and the other partner is in the second group that wants minimal information. In these cases, it is fine to have a double standard of disclosure. One partner will give the other much more information about outside relationships, because that is what makes them most comfortable, and they will in turn give their partner a very small amount of information, because their partner doesn't want to hear very much.

If you feel a strong need to "confess" everything that is going on with your outside partners, and your primary partner makes it clear that they do not want to know all the details, talk to a friend or a therapist instead of using your partner as a sounding board or a support group. This does not mean that you should lie to your partner or omit significant events, important changes in your feelings, the status of an outside relationship, or the development of a new sexual or romantic relationship. It just means you should use discretion in how much to talk about your outside partners and how much detail to provide about those relationships. Your partner's comfort level is much more important than you having a constant outlet for your polyamorous thoughts, feelings, and activities.

You may find that you feel very comfortable with a certain level of disclosure in one situation but feel a need for much more (or much less) information with another partner, because of the complex constellation of different feelings and fears engendered by particular partners and relationships. My best advice is to proceed slowly and with caution, and don't hesitate to modify your agreements, as your feelings may change over time.

An even more vexing problem is that many people guess wrong about how much they need to know. They demand a lot of information and ask lots of questions but they painfully discover that much of what they hear causes such distress that they wish they never asked. This makes your partner very reluctant to disclose much in the future because when they answered your questions this time, you freaked out and this led to endless processing and drama.

For example:

Joan made the mistake of asking her lesbian partner Mary if her new lover Tina was good in bed. This led to a discussion where it came to light that Tina in fact had some specific sexual skills that Joan had not developed. Joan was devastated and became very insecure about her desirability as a lover.

Sam asked his wife Maya what she liked most about her new boyfriend. She replied that he was very intellectual and they had interesting talks about philosophy and politics. Sam became despondent and felt convinced that his wife thought he was stupid and boring, despite her repeated protestations that this was completely untrue.

It is often difficult to know which pieces of information will be helpful and which will exacerbate jealousy and anxieties. Most people learn by trial and error what level of disclosure and what kind of information they really want, and which will only cause pain. As one woman said to her husband, "If your new girlfriend gives better blowjobs than I do, I'm happy for you, but please don't tell me about it, because it will only make me feel insecure. And if she's a brilliant genius with an IQ off the charts, please keep that to yourself, too, because it will only make me feel inadequate."

Another area of conflict is not just how much you want to know but when you want to know it. Take this brief quiz about the timing of disclosure. Should you tell your partner about a new person in your life:

a) before you have sex with another person?

b) when you first begin to "court" a potential new partner, when you first flirt or exchange phone numbers or send each other emails?

c) when you first develop an attraction towards someone but before you ask them for a date or reveal your interest to them?

d) just before the first date?

e) right after the first date?

f) after you first have sex with the new person?

g) when you decide to have an ongoing relationship with them?

h) any of the above

If you said h), you would be right, as couples can decide on any of these parameters, depending on their individual needs. There is no right or wrong way to do this, as each person and each relationship varies in what agreements provide the right comfort level. The goal is to balance each partner and each relationship's optimal level of disclosure with each partner's need for privacy and agency. This can be difficult and require some compromise.

As in many poly situations, there seems to be a gender difference in the ideal timing of disclosure. As usual, these are gross generalizations which are not true for all men or all women, but there is enough of a trend to warrant a mention. Women are more likely to want to be told as soon as their partner becomes romantically interested in someone else, even if the partner hasn't even approached that person yet and doesn't have a clue if their interest is reciprocated. Many women feel deceived and betrayed if their partner doesn't mention anything until there is a courtship underway and a date planned. I have heard many women say things like, "How could you keep this from me?" "Why didn't you tell me you were emailing her and calling her?" "I knew you were being secretive about something!" "I can't believe you told her you were attracted to her and made a date with her before telling me about it!" These comments usually leave the man baffled and defensive, convinced he has done nothing wrong because no lies have been told and there has been full disclosure before the first date. Often the exasperated man will say things like, "But I haven't even touched her yet!" "We haven't even had coffee!" "We've just been emailing, there's nothing going on!" However, because many women are much more concerned about their partner's level of emotional intimacy than about whether they have actually had a date or had sex, the fact that some courtship has occurred without their knowledge makes them feel excluded and betrayed.

Other women have a different threshold for disclosure, and just want to know about an outside partner before any sexual activity is initiated. This creates problems for many men, because they often have no idea when or if sex will occur, because they see that decision as largely resting with the woman. One man explained, "I met a woman at a poly event, and we exchanged phone numbers. She called me and invited me to have coffee. I went on four dates with her but each time I wasn't sure if she was interested in me romantically or just wanted to be friends. There was nothing physical except an innocent hug hello. I told my wife that I was seeing this woman but that it was platonic. On the fifth date, she invited me over to her house for dinner, we had some wine, and she invited me to go to bed and have sex. I told my wife later that night and she went ballistic, saying I lied because I had said we were just friends. But we *were* just friends until that moment that she asked me to go to bed with her."

Some couples make an agreement that they will tell each other if they are attracted to someone or have "sexual intentions" towards someone new, even if they aren't sure if anything will come of it. However, one man found this requirement untenable, explaining, "I meet women every day that I find sexually attractive, and whom I would sleep with given the opportunity, but most of the time nothing is going to happen. I am not going to tell my partner every time I meet a sexually attractive woman, or I would be freaking her out for no reason nine times out of ten. Why make a big deal out of an attraction and put my partner through some anxiety and asking me a million questions about my intentions and plans, when it is just a nice fantasy and nothing is likely to come of it?" Still other men feel that if they tell their partner about a potential sexual partner, they will feel foolish if it doesn't actually pan out. One man said, "It's bad enough to be sexually rejected when you are trying to date someone. On top of that, I don't want to have to go back to my partner and tell them they got all jealous for no reason because this woman doesn't want to sleep with me anyway!"

Conversely, many men would rather not hear about anything until there actually is a relationship and it looks like this will be an ongoing thing. Most men want to know immediately if their partner has had sex with someone else, but until and unless sex takes place, they don't want to hear about the courtship. Ben said that his partner Jennifer frequently corresponded with both women and men by email that she connected with on dating websites. Many of them never got past the email stage to even a phone call. Ben told her to stop telling him every time she was interested in someone. He explained that it made him anxious, as he was psychologically preparing himself to deal with her having a new relationship, and then usually nothing happened. He told her to just let him know if she actually had sex with someone, and then he would handle whatever feelings came up for him.

For some men, there is no need to know anything until it is clear that the outside relationship will affect them in some way. One man explained, "My wife travels on business and goes to conferences, and often has fun sexual adventures when she is out of town. I really don't need to know about these one-time flings unless she really feels like sharing or if she feels it will bring us closer together to tell me about it. It's over and she will never see the person again, so why should I grill her about the whole thing? However, if she really connects with someone and is going to correspond with them or plans to be involved with them again in the future, then I want to know that something is going on."

Because the issue of disclosure is so complex and has such potential to create crises and drama, I encourage you to come up with your own individual list of what information you need, and when you need to know it, so you can communicate this clearly to your partners and negotiate a mutually satisfactory agreement.

As an example of one experienced poly person's disclosure needs, here's mine. This list is not intended to be exhaustive, nor to serve as a model for anyone else; it's simply one person's list of need-to-know information. If my partner is involved with another person, I want to know four things:

- *Have you been involved in a sexual situation with this person, or do you intend to become sexual with him or her?* I deliberately use the term "sexual situation" rather than saying "Did you have sex with him or her?" This is because each person has their own definition of sex and I have seen many, many misunderstandings over whether someone actually had sex with an outside partner or not. You may recall former President Bill Clinton's vehement denial "I did not have sex with that woman," because he had received fellatio to orgasm on numerous occasions but did not have vaginal intercourse (except with a cigar). I have heard similar statements from many people that they "didn't really have sex," because they "just fooled around," or "just had cunnilingus," or "we were only making out", or "she just gave me a hand job," or "it was mutual masturbation, not sex," etc. Usually in these situations the partner feels manipulated, deceived, and betrayed, even though there may not have been an overt lie so much as a different definition of what constitutes sex. As a result, I prefer the more generic term "sexual situation," as it includes anything that could remotely be defined as sexual activity. Asking my partner this question means, "Did you do anything physical with this person that you would not do with a platonic friend?" In my definition, this includes kissing, touching of any part of the body that could be construed as sexual (breasts, buttocks, clitoris, vagina, penis, anus), making out, getting naked together, using sex toys, having oral sex, manual sex, mutual masturbation, and vaginal or anal intercourse.

I want to know if my partner has been in a sexual situation with someone or if they intend to do so, because to me that is a significant piece of news, something new and different going on in my partner's life that may affect me, and I want to know about it. This is true even if it is a casual, one-time sexual experience with someone they will never see again. I still want to be aware of it and know what is going on. I don't need to know whether they made out or whether they had oral sex or whether they had vaginal or anal intercourse – that is Too Much Information for me and will only fill my head with images of the delightful sexual activities they enjoyed, trigger my own insecurities about my desirability, and convince me that I don't measure up when compared to this new person. I know that for many poly people, having this information is reassuring and having their partner share this feels intimate and is a bonding experience. For some couples, it can create what is sometimes called the "sexual spillover effect," in that talking about their outside sexual experiences together makes them appreciate each other more and is sexually arousing. For me, it has the opposite effect, so I just want to know if there was a sexual situation or if there is an intention of becoming sexual with this person.

- *Is this an ongoing romantic or sexual relationship or is it over?* I want my partner to tell me if this was a one-time thing, or whether there is an intention to have a relationship with this person for the foreseeable future. Clearly, if it's over, it is much easier to accept it and move on. If it is ongoing, it requires a lot more from me to manage my feelings about it and to work with my partner to make it a successful relationship.

   If it is ongoing, what is the status of this new relationship? In order for me to accommodate this new relationship and know what to expect, I need to know what the nature of this relationship is and what role this new person will play in my partner's life. Is this a casual sex partner or play partner? Is this a "fuck buddy" or "friend with benefits?" Is this a lover or ongoing secondary relationship? Or do you have serious feelings for this new partner, and do you consider this potentially primary?

- *How will this affect me? I* want to know whether this new relationship, whether casual or serious, will mean that my partner will have less time for me, whether this means I will be getting less attention or less sex, or whether it will just make it more complicated scheduling dates because there is another person's schedule to take into consideration. Does this new person have an STD that I need to be concerned about or that may influence me to change my sexual practices with my partner? Has this new relationship changed my partner's feelings for me, or altered my role or status in their life? Often in the beginning it is difficult to answer these questions accurately, because it is too soon to tell. I expect my partner to keep me informed of new developments as they happen, such as whether their feelings for me are beginning to change as a result of this outside relationship. However, I also feel it is my responsibility to bring this up from time to time and voice my questions and concerns, rather than put all the responsibility for disclosure on my partner.

- *Timing of the disclosure.* When do I need to know that my partner is getting involved with someone? My bottom line is that I need to hear something from them as soon as possible after they have been in a sexual situation with a new person for the first time. Ideally, I would like them to tell me the next time I see them after this new sexual relationship has happened, but I am happy to give them some "wiggle room" in the interests of my partner picking a time and place to tell me that feels comfortable to them. Once my partner informs me that they have started having sex with someone new, they don't need to tell me again about the fact that they are having a sexual relationship with this person. I will assume that sex will continue to be a part of that relationship unless they tell me the relationship is no longer sexual.

While sex is the dividing line at which I really need some disclosure, I generally prefer that my partner tell me they are interested in someone else at the point where it seems clear that the relationship is moving from platonic to romantic. Since this shift is not always obvious and sometimes happens quickly, I'm comfortable with the reality that sometimes I won't hear anything until this change has already occurred, and the relationship has already become sexual. I prefer to hear about my partner's intentions when the courtship is first starting, because then it comes as no surprise when a sexual relationship is initiated, and I am more likely to handle it with a minimum of stress.

If the relationship goes on for a significant period of time, I am likely to have a few additional questions about what the relationship means to my partner, and what my partner receives in this other relationship. I am likely to ask those questions not so much because I need disclosure of this information. Rather, because I feel connected to my partner, I want to know about the important things going on in their life, including relationships, and have an understanding of why this is significant for them. If my partner got very involved in an activity such as a new job, a political organization, volunteering in some kind of community service, or a hobby, I would want to understand what is compelling about that activity and how it fits into their life. Similarly, I would like to know what an outside relationship means to them and how it enhances their life. Admittedly, this is really none of my business, and I don't really need to know for my emotional well-being. But because I care about my partner and want to know them better, I am very curious and want to know all about what is going on with them. They have the right to tell me if they want more privacy around this and I will respect their wishes.

This list reflects my own personal needs and evolved out of my life experience and relationship history, and should not be construed as a template for anyone else's relationship agreements. I include it here to illustrate some of the possible needs that polyamorous people may have for disclosure of outside relationships. I encourage you to develop you own disclosure agreements based on your unique constellation of family history, past relationship trauma, personality traits, and security needs.

What Are You Asking For?

The second most common communication problem experienced by polyamorous couples is lack of clarity about whether the goal of your communication is action-oriented or not. What you are asking for? Are you expressing feelings? Or are you requesting a change in behavior, or a change in your relationship agreements?

A typical problem occurs when one partner is experiencing some kind of distress over their partner's outside relationships. They express their feelings and their partner misconstrues the goal of that communication. Do they just want to express their feelings and receive support and acknowledgement, or are they asking for a change in their partner's behavior or a change in their relationship agreements?

For example:

Melissa and John are a bisexual couple in a long-term, committed relationship. John also has a relationship with Ricardo. Their agreement is that John can spend two weeknights with Ricardo each week. He negotiates with

Melissa to spend the weekend with Ricardo for the first time. She agrees, knowing it will be difficult for her, but trying to stretch herself to allow this because she knows it is important to both John and Ricardo. Melissa plans to spend one night of the weekend with her girlfriend Rhonda, but Rhonda's baby gets sick with the flu at the last minute so Melissa spends the weekend alone. When John returns home on Monday morning, he thanks her for her willingness to accept this arrangement, reiterating that this has been really great to have this quality time with Ricardo. Melissa breaks down crying and tells him how hard it was for her and how she couldn't sleep and had bouts of jealousy and despair all weekend. She tells him how angry it made her thinking about him being with someone else all weekend and leaving her home alone. John becomes defensive, saying, "But you said it was okay, and now you're changing your mind. What do you expect me to do?" She keeps trying to express her feelings, but John is so busy defending himself that he can't give her the validation she needs. She just wants support, but he mistakenly believes she is telling him he should not have spent the weekend with Ricardo and that he cannot do so again. Both feel hurt and misunderstood, and nothing is resolved.

This type of communication breakdown is very typical of polyamorous relationships. The best approach is to remember to meta-communicate, as discussed earlier in this chapter. In the above example, Melissa could have immediately communicated to John that she was not asking for any change in the agreement or in his behavior, but just wanted to be heard and for him to acknowledge that she had done something that was really hard for her. Or she could have asked him to hold her and reconnect, to re-establish a feeling of intimacy after being separated for a few days. Or John could have asked her whether the weekend had been tolerable or whether she wanted to change the agreement. It is often difficult to metacommunicate when emotions are running high and people are experiencing a stressful polyamorous situation. However, if you can clarify whether you want to express your feelings, be comforted, create intimacy, or if you are asking for some specific action or change, many arguments and hurt feelings can be avoided.

Now that you have learned and practiced these crucial communication skills, you have all the tools you need to address the most challenging aspect of open relationships: jealousy. Part Three is divided into three chapters which will help you understand jealousy and provides two different approaches for managing and defusing jealousy.

PART THREE

Unmasking the Green-Eyed Monster: Managing Jealousy In Open Relationships

6 Why Are We Jealous?

For most people, the biggest obstacle to creating successful and satisfying open relationships is jealousy. Despite how enlightened we think we are, most of us experience jealousy if our spouse or lover has a sexual relationship with someone else.

A few rare individuals never experience jealousy. They are either more highly evolved than the rest of us mere mortals, or else they are pathologically out of touch with their feelings. I advise clients to treat jealousy as a given: assume that it will occur, and be prepared with strategies to successfully address it and minimize the distress.

Of course, jealousy is present in our lives literally from birth, and not just in romantic relationships. In thinking back on your life, you may recall experiencing jealousy in many childhood situations:

- Your parents were busy with their work or other activities and didn't give you as much time and attention as you wanted.

- The birth of a new sibling suddenly took all the attention away from you and focused it on the new baby.

- A parent seemed to like another sibling more, or another sibling was better-behaved, did better in school, or was more successful socially.

- You didn't get picked for the football team but other friends made the team.

- Your best friend started spending more time with another friend.

- A friend became more popular than you and was invited into a "cool" clique.

- Other friends seemed to get more dates than you do.

- A friend got better grades and got into a better college.

In adulthood, some of these situations may provoke intense jealousy:

- Your neighbor has a nicer house than you or buys a very expensive car.

- Your co-worker gets the promotion you applied for.

- Your boss refuses to give you a raise but gives one to another co-worker.

- Your best friend marries someone with a lot of money or who is much better-looking than your spouse.

- Your partner spends too much time at work, on sports, on the computer, or on hobbies, and not enough time with you.

- Your partner would rather drink or use drugs than spend time with you.

- Your neighbor's kid gets into Harvard and your kid is an unemployed pothead.

- Your friends all have grandchildren but you have none.

- Your partner seems more loyal and committed to their children from a previous marriage than to you.

Many situations in childhood and previous adult experiences provoke intense jealousy. As a result, when we experience jealousy in a romantic relationship we may be triggering traumatic events from our past and projecting those feelings onto the present situation. This may explain in part why we can feel so out of control when jealousy strikes, since it is not just about the current situation but about very painful experiences in the past.

Everyone from philosophers to psychologists to evolutionary biologists have weighed in with theories about the origins of jealousy and why it exists. While theories abound, there has not been enough scientific study of jealousy to come to any conclusions. However, each theory may have some kernel of truth and be useful to you in understanding how jealousy affects you and your relationships.

Freud's Theory of Jealousy

Sigmund Freud, the inventor of modern psychiatry, believed that jealousy was rooted in the Oedipal conflict. He posited that every child falls in love with the opposite-sex parent, and becomes insanely jealous of the same-sex parent because the child eventually realizes that the object of their affection is in love with the other parent. According to Freud, the devastating experience of loss and betrayal in this triangle forms the basis of the primal experience of jealousy in adulthood, when the man is faced with the potential loss of his partner's love to another man. He hypothesized that this sense of loss creates a life-long insecurity that can be triggered whenever we are faced with any real or imagined competition for our spouse's or partner's romantic attention. This is a very heterosexual view of jealousy, and the Oedipal interpretation does not explain why same-sex couples experience jealousy just as intensely as heterosexuals.

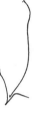

Freud identified four major components of jealousy. First, he believed, we experience grief, the terrible pain of actually losing or being afraid of losing someone we love. Second, we are flooded with the very distressing realization that we cannot have everything we want in life. Third, we are gripped with feelings of enmity towards the successful rival who has won the love of our partner or whom we fear will succeed in stealing our partner. Fourth, we turn our anger on ourselves in a belief that our own inadequacies as a partner will cause our partner to leave us. So as you can see, Freud viewed jealousy as a nightmare driven by our most primal fears of inferiority, loss, and abandonment. In his construct, jealousy triggers our most intense emotions: terror of being rejected and alone, despair at the realization that we can't have what we desire most, rage at a rival for trying to steal our partner's love and attention, self-blame and loathing for being inadequate and "losing" a competition with a hated competitor.

"Darwinian" Theories of Jealousy

Evolutionary biologists have taken a somewhat different approach to the origins of jealousy and have assumed that it serves an evolutionary purpose, that it developed because it was useful in the survival of the species. They believe that jealousy in humans is hard-wired because it is evolution's way of getting us to pay attention to a potential threat to the family unit. In the days of cavemen and -women, if a man and woman had a baby, the mother and child were somewhat dependent on the male (during pregnancy and during the child's first years) to hunt for food and protect them from predators (including other men). If the male ran off with another female, it decreased the chances that the child would survive to adulthood and reproduce, and continue the human species, which is the main goal of evolution. Similarly, if the woman ran off with another man, the abandoned male would not be able to reproduce. In this scenario, jealousy served approximately the same purpose as a car alarm: an early warning system. The more jealous someone was, the more likely they would notice signs that the partner was sexually involved with another partner and was considering defecting to another mate. The more jealous partner would be more likely to take action to intervene to try to prevent this outcome. Since this trait had a survival value, people who were more jealous were more likely to reproduce their genetic material and therefore those traits would be accentuated over many generations.

Some biologists have presented evidence that women tend to be more jealous than men. They hypothesize that a woman and her children were much more vulnerable to death or hunger due to the male's abandoning the family for another mate. They theorize that if the woman left for another man, she would take her children with her and they would be likely to be protected by and provided for by the new mate, and likely to survive to adulthood and reproduce. Thus the male did not have nearly as strong an evolutionary reason for jealousy to become pronounced.

However, many other people have presented evidence that men are just as jealous as women, but that they experience and express it differently. Women are more likely to internalize jealousy as fear and despair while men are more likely to project it outward as anger towards their partner or the person they see as a rival. Many women tend to experience jealousy very intensely and can become incapacitated and almost paralyzed by fear, depression, and self-hatred. Men, on the other hand, may not experience jealousy internally quite as intensely, but instead tend to act it out through tantrums, threats, and even violence. These are broad generalizations and are certainly not true for all men or all women, but manifest often enough that some general trends can be seen.

Charles Darwin himself pointed out that men's jealousy tend to be focused on their female partner having sex with another man, while women's jealousy is more likely to focus on their male partner developing an intimate or committed relationship with another woman. He hypothesized that there is an evolutionary purpose for these gender-specific manifestations of jealousy. Modern sociobiologists have elaborated on Darwin's theory. They believe that the male is more concerned about sex because if his mate has sex with another man, she may become pregnant by someone else and he will be supporting and raising someone else's children. Conversely, the woman is more jealous of the man developing a committed relationship because she fears he will invest his time, energy, protection, and resources in another woman, and she herself will have less resources and safety if she has to share the male's resources with another woman and her children.

According to this theory, both male and female jealousy have the same evolutionary goal, to protect the pair bond in order to maximize the chances of the couple having children and staying together long enough for those children to survive to adulthood.

What Current Research Tells Us About Jealousy

Dr. Ayala Pines is a psychologist who has spent her entire career researching jealousy, and has written several books on the subject. She has studied every aspect of what makes people jealous, why certain triggers affect some people and not others, and ways to manage and reduce jealousy. Although her books were written for monogamous, heterosexual married couples, her research is useful for polyamorous people as well.

She identifies two kinds of jealousy, acute and chronic. She believes that acute jealousy is very similar to post-traumatic stress disorder (PTSD), in that it almost always manifests with the same core symptoms: intrusion, constriction, and hyperarousal. "Intrusion" refers to being bombarded with intrusive thoughts and feelings about the painful situation (usually your partner being with another partner) that are difficult to stop, remembering and re-experiencing images of the traumatic events over and over, having flashbacks, ruminating on the problem, and becoming obsessed with painful thoughts about it. "Constriction" refers to feeling estranged from your life and the people around you, feeling alone and unloved, losing interest in your usual activities, and feeling no pleasure. "Hyperarousal" refers to the experience of hypervigilance, of being very anxious about your relationship and about whatever your partner is doing with someone else, feeling agitated and irritable, unable to relax; it often includes insomnia. Acute jealousy is usually related to a specific situation, like your partner showing interest in getting involved with someone new, or an outside relationship becoming more serious than it was before. It usually comes on suddenly in response to a traumatic event or disclosure, and can be extremely intense, but often begins to subside in a relatively short time, from a few hours to a few days.

Chronic jealousy is when someone feels jealous all or most of the time, regardless of whether there is a specific situation that is currently triggering the experience of jealousy. Dr. Pines' research indicates that some people have a tendency to be much more jealous than others, either due to their own temperament and life experience or due to ongoing behaviors of their partner which create insecurity. Intrusion, constriction, and hyperarousal are usually present in chronic jealousy, but are much less intense than in acute jealousy.

Dr. Pines's theory is that your experience of jealousy grows out of your own life history both in childhood and in previous intimate relationships, combined with the history of your current relationship. As a result, each person has their own unique jealousy profile. She says that whatever brought two people together as a couple is the exact thing that will shape your jealousy experience. To get to the core of your jealousy, think back to what attracted you to your partner in the first place. What is the most valuable thing you receive from this relationship that caused you to fall in love with your partner? That is likely to be the thing you are most afraid of losing, and the fear of that loss is usually the spark that ignites the jealousy attack. If great sex is the "glue" that most strongly connects you with your partner, you will be most likely to feel most jealous of the sexual aspect of your partner's outside relationships. If companionship and emotional intimacy are the most precious parts of your relationship, you will feel most threatened by any indication that the outside relationship also provides friendship and emotional closeness for your partner. If intellectual rapport and lively discussions of politics or ideas are central to your relationship, an outside partner who is smart and interesting will feel most threatening. If shared activities are important in your relationship, an outside relationship that "invades" that activity will trigger intense jealousy (i.e.: you and your partner love to go backpacking and the new lover also loves backpacking).

According to Dr. Pines's research, temperament and personality also play a big role in how jealous we are. She argues that the more confident and secure a person feels in their own life, their abilities, and their relationship, the less jealous they will be in any given situation where an insecure person would become much more jealous. The people who are most vulnerable to jealousy are those who have low self-esteem and are very emotionally dependent on their love relationship to give meaning to their lives and make them feel good about themselves. Her advice: anything you can do to increase your self-esteem, sense of personal security, resilience, and self-sufficiency will make you a less jealous person. However, even very strong, independent people with high self-esteem can become very jealous if their relationship is not secure or their partner does not provide them with adequate love and reassurance.

She suggests that there are five cardinal fears triggered by jealousy and that for each person, one will be primary. She identifies them as:

- Fear of abandonment ("He's going to leave me for someone else")

- Losing face and losing status in our community ("How could she humiliate me by telling our friends about sleeping with him?")

- Betrayal ("I just can't believe he would hurt me like this!")

- Competitiveness and fear of our own inadequacy: ("I wonder if her new lover is better in bed than me!")

- Envy towards our partner's other partner ("If only I was as attractive/smart/successful/rich/etc as he is!")

It behooves each person to look carefully at all five and try to discern which one is most distressing to you, as this can help you understand and manage your jealousy. If you discover that you are most shaken up by fears of abandonment, you will know it is time to work on your own sense of security and confidence as well as ask your partner for reassurance and support to demonstrate their commitment to stay in the relationship. If you find that you are most concerned with the "public relations" aspect of feeling somehow humiliated by other people knowing that your partner has another lover, you can either ask your partner to be more discreet and keep things private, or you can learn not to be as worried about what others may think of you and your partner. If you find that competitiveness or envy of the outside partner is a primary jealousy trigger for you, it is important for you to boost your self-esteem through counseling, affirmations, or activities that make you feel good about yourself.

Ralph Hupka, a cross-cultural psychologist, has done extensive studies of jealousy in a wide variety of cultures around the world, and has found fascinating differences in the experience and manifestations of jealousy depending on cultural expectations. His research shows that some cultures encourage jealousy and condone jealous behavior much more than others. He found that all cultures that strongly encourage jealousy have four characteristics in common:

- A strong emphasis on property rights, in relation to material possessions, land, and "ownership" and control of spouse and children

- Social codes that make sex a scarce resource and restrict access to sex with many rules and taboos

- Emphasis on having many children and specifically on known paternity of those children, and

- Strong emphasis on marriage for economic survival and social status, more so than for love and companionship.

Cultures that emphasize those values tend to institutionalize and condone jealous behavior and predispose individuals to experience and act out intense jealousy if they believe their mate is having an outside relationship. According to Hupka, these attitudes and behaviors are largely learned, due to the cues and cultural norms in each society. Conversely, he studied other cultures where jealousy is not given such emphasis and not encouraged, and in those cultures there is much less jealous behavior. This research underlines the possibility that jealousy may not be so innate after all, and that if it can be learned, it can be unlearned.

Another Approach

As a counselor working with polyamorous clients and as a polyamorous woman for nearly forty years, I have my own theory about jealousy. I have come to believe that jealousy is a normal, natural response that serves a valid purpose. It comes up when we feel threatened with loss of something precious to us, and alerts us to pay attention to our relationships to make sure they are safe and sound.

Like a smoke alarm that may go off when you only burned the toast, jealousy may sometimes be an overreaction. When the smoke alarm goes off, it makes you pay attention. Once you're sure the problem is only burned toast and the house is not on fire, you can relax and forget about it. However, if the house is on fire, or your relationship is in danger, you can take whatever steps are needed to strengthen your relationship and fix whatever is causing the problem.

In an open relationship, it is important to recognize that any new outside relationship is a potential threat to the survival of your relationship. The emphasis should be on the word "potential." A new relationship is not a threat *per se,* but any new relationship has the potential to disrupt, destabilize, or destroy your relationship. Anyone who has been in an open relationship or been around polyamorous people for any length of time has seen situations where a new relationship did in fact destroy an existing relationship. (Of course, this situation is also common in nominally monogamous relationships!) So it is foolhardy to make believe that this could never happen to you.

Instead, make jealousy your protective ally, and pay attention to jealous feelings, as they can encourage you to look closely at what is going on in your relationship and continue to assess whether there is cause for concern or whether you can turn down the jealousy alarm.

The Four Prerequisite Conditions for Jealousy

Remember that jealousy occurs in all kinds of situations, not just in romantic relationships. Jealousy is a reaction to feeling threatened with the potential loss of something that is valuable to us: the love or loyalty of a friend, lover, or family member, the quality of a relationship, time, sexual access, a job, possessions, wealth, our status or position in our family or community, or our health and abilities. For jealousy to exist, usually all four of these conditions need to be present:

1) You want something very badly that you don't have, a valuable resource such as a job, money, status, or a relationship,

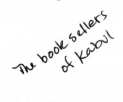

OR you want time, attention, affection, love, loyalty, priority, or sexual attention from a particular person in your life (spouse, lover, friend, parent, child, boss, etc.)

OR you already have that resource that you desire (any of the above) but you fear losing it to someone else.

2) Another person wants that same resource, such as the same job, the same partner, love of a parent, sex with your partner, a business opportunity, etc.

3) You believe yourself to be in direct competition with that other person to get what you want, and you believe there is a scarcity of this resource and that there is not enough for both of you to get what you want.

4) You believe that if push comes to shove, you will lose this contest and your competitor will win out. In other words, you will be compared to your rival, and you will be found inadequate, and they will be seen as superior and/or more desirable, and they will walk away with the prize, whatever that is.

A good exercise to try when you are feeling jealous is to go through these four conditions and ask yourself if all four are met. If less than all four are true, your jealousy is unfounded and you can take steps to get it under control.

Say you see someone flirting with your partner at a party, and you suddenly feel jealous. If you look at the first condition listed above, you will see that this condition is met, because you do in fact already possess the precious resource (you are in a committed relationship which is valuable to you), and you fear losing it to someone else (the person flirting with your partner).

If you look at the second condition, you cannot say with any certainty that it is true, as you do not know whether this other person wants what you have. You can't immediately know their motives for flirting with your partner: they may be just flirting for fun, or to manipulate their own partner, or to impress someone else, or to validate their self-esteem, or because they think your partner can help them get a job or be useful in some other way. It is entirely possible that they are flirting because they hope to sleep with your partner and even to steal them away from you, but you can't jump to that conclusion based on the current evidence you have.

Looking at the third condition, you cannot know if that is true, for two reasons: 1) You do not know if this person intends to try to get involved with your partner, or even whether your partner is even the least bit interested in this person — they may just be enjoying getting some attention, or being polite. 2) You have not established that there is a shortage of this resource, as it is possible that if your partner does get involved with this person, there may still be plenty of love and time and attention for you, and you may not experience deprivation.

If you look at the fourth condition, you will see that this is also not objectively true, for three reasons: 1) you don't know if you are in any kind of competition with this other person or being compared to them. Even if your partner does get involved with them, they may receive very different things from that relationship than they enjoy in your relationship, so there would be no reason to compare the two. 2) You have no reason to believe that if you are compared, that you will be somehow found wanting. Look carefully at your own insecurities to see why you feel this other person would be seen by your partner as more desirable and why you fear your partner will abandon you for them. This will give you strong clues about what makes you most jealous. Are you seeing this new person as more physically attractive, smarter, more interesting, funnier, more affluent than yourself? 3) There is no reason to believe that your partner will choose this person over you. This is your own insecurity talking and creating panic inside you, fearing that your partner will abandon you for anyone who shows a little interest in them.

So as you can see, often our jealousy does not stand up to scrutiny when faced with the reality of the situation. As in the example above, you may be able to understand your jealousy more fully by going through this process of checking to see if it meets all four of these conditions. Often you can see that one or more of these conditions are not met, and as a result you can allow your jealousy to subside naturally, as it is not founded in a real threat to the stability or your relationship but rather on irrational fears.

What if you feel jealous and on going through these four conditions you discover that all four are met?

For example:

Tania and Ross are a married couple, and Tania has had an outside "secondary" relationship for a year with Jack.

Ross has become extremely jealous because in the past few months, Tania is spending more and more time with Jack, and is giving Ross less time and attention. She frequently is "too tired" for sex with Ross, which is a big change from their usually robust sexual relationship. She has started going on trips with Jack, saying he is "more fun and adventurous," and has started to complain the she and Ross "just don't have chemistry anymore." Tania has told Ross that she feels very conflicted because Jack wants a monogamous relationship and wants her to leave Ross and marry him.

As you can see, this situation meets all four conditions for jealousy and any reasonable person would feel very threatened because their relationship is in grave danger. Condition one is met: Ross has a relationship that he values very much, and fears losing Tania to Jack. Condition two is met: Jack also wants what Ross has, and is pressuring Tania to leave Ross. Condition three is also met: Because Jack wants Tania to be monogamous with him, he and Ross cannot both get what they want. Condition four is also true: Tania is giving every sign that she is comparing Ross to Jack and that she sees Ross as inadequate, and that in a direct competition, Ross is in danger of losing Tania to Jack.

In this situation, jealousy is completely rational and is necessary for the survival of the relationship. It forces Ross and Tania to look closely at their relationship and work to repair their level of closeness as well as the physical intimacy that they seem to have neglected. If they are committed to their relationship and willing to work on it, they may be able to resolve whatever problems led Tania to become so heavily invested in an outside relationship that she would consider leaving her husband. Sometimes it is too late and the partner has already emotionally abandoned the primary relationship, and has decided to pursue the new relationship at the expense of the old one.

If you find your jealousy is rational and reflects a real threat to your relationship, it's time to seek couples counseling or some form of support to rebuild your level of trust and intimacy. Express your feelings as calmly and clearly as you can to your partner and don't allow them to trivialize or discount your fears. A counselor or therapist who has expertise in open relationships can help you and your partner see the situation as objectively as possible and identify what steps are necessary to get back on track.

7 Unmasking Jealousy

What Exactly Is Jealousy?

We tend to think of jealousy as a single emotion, but actually it is a whole bundle of feelings that tend to get lumped together. Jealousy can manifest as anger, fear, hurt, betrayal, anxiety, agitation, sadness, paranoia, depression, loneliness, envy, coveting, self-loathing, feeling powerless, feeling inadequate, feeling excluded.

It often helps to identify what is the exact mix of feelings you experience when you feel jealous. Demystifying the exact components of your jealousy can be a giant step towards understanding and resolving it. Is it always the same for you or does the mix change from time to time depending on circumstances?

For instance, one woman figured out that her jealousy was about 50% fear, 20% anger, 20% feeling powerless and 10% feeling betrayed. However, when she asked her partner for reassurance and affection, and he provided it, the anger and betrayal disappeared. Then her jealousy was much more manageable, because most of what was left was fear and she could express those feelings more easily to her partner and resolve them.

It is crucial to understand what jealousy is and what it is about. Jealousy provokes some of our deepest fears — fear of the unknown and of change, fear of losing power or control in a relationship, fear of scarcity and of loss, and fear of abandonment. First, it triggers our own insecurity about our worthiness, anxiety about being adequate as a lover, and doubts about our desirability.

Second, it taps into our deepest fears about our partner's integrity, loyalty, and commitment to us, making us doubt ourselves for trusting them and wonder if they will betray us.

For every jealous feeling, there is an emotion behind the jealousy that is much more significant than the jealousy itself. Recognizing those fears and unmet needs is the key to unmasking jealousy and taking away its power. Jealousy is just the finger pointing at the fears and needs we are afraid to face. When jealousy kicks in, it is the ancient reptilian part of our brain going into a "fight or flight" response because we feel that our very survival is threatened.

A "Jealousy Intervention" Exercise

When you feel jealous, an immediate intervention can be helpful. Try this exercise: Ask yourself the following questions and write the answers down:

"What exactly am I feeling?"

"Where do these feelings come from?"

"What is it that I am really afraid of?"

 What do I need to make this situation safe for me?"

"What can I do for myself right now, and what do I need to ask for from my partner, friends, and support system?"

 "What is the worst thing that could happen and how likely is that to happen?"

If you are feeling too incapacitated by a jealousy attack to go through this entire exercise, an abbreviated version can be useful. Just take a few deep breaths and answer these three questions verbally or in writing, whichever you can manage at the moment:

"What am I feeling?"

"Where is the source of my pain?"

"What do I need?"

Unlearning Core Beliefs That Inevitably Generate Jealousy

Three core beliefs about relationships are very deeply entrenched in our society, and these beliefs are guaranteed to create jealousy even in the most well-adjusted people. Most of us have absorbed these beliefs without even realizing it. Identifying and dismantling these beliefs in our "heart of hearts" is the single most effective way to short-circuit jealousy. Ask yourself how much of you believes each of these three statements. Is it 90% of yourself that believes them? 50%? Notice which belief is most entrenched in your mind, and more importantly, your gut, and which one you are least attached to:

Core Belief #1

If my partner really loved me, (s)he wouldn't have any desire for a sexual relationship with anyone else.

This belief sees any interest your partner has in anyone else as a direct reflection of how much (s)he loves you. It's a quantitative view of love which equates the amount of love with the ability to be interested in having another partner. When you break it down, this is as absurd as saying that a couple that gives birth to a second child must not love their first child or they couldn't possibly have any interest in having a second one, or that you couldn't possibly love your good friend if you are interested in making new friends.

Core Belief #2

If my partner were happy with me, and if I were a good partner/spouse/lover/etc., my partner would be so satisfied that (s)he wouldn't want to get involved with anyone else.

This belief is even more insidious. With the first belief you can at least blame it on your partner for not loving you enough. This belief says that if your partner is interested in someone else, it's your fault for not being the perfect lover or spouse and your relationship must be a failure. If you truly believe that your lover could only be interested in another partner because you're inadequate, you can see how this belief is certain to generate jealousy.

Core Belief #3

It's just not possible to love more than one person at the same time.

This belief is built on the "scarcity economy of love," the belief that love is a finite resource, there is only so much to go around, and there is never enough. Therefore, if my partner gives any love to anyone else, that necessarily means that there's less for me. Because most people already feel there are some areas in their relationship where they are not getting enough of something (time, love, affection, sex, support, commitment), they are fearful that they will receive even less if their partner gets involved with additional partners.

Because each of these beliefs is connected to a very primal fear, they take time and effort to mitigate. The first belief expresses a deep fear that you are not loved and will be abandoned. The second taps into our insecurities and the fear that we are not adequate or deserving of love, and the third is a fear of deprivation and being starved for love and attention. So have compassion for yourself and your partner(s) as you work with these beliefs and gradually replace them with beliefs that support your desire to embrace open relationships. Try on these new beliefs instead and see how they feel to you.

New Core Belief #1

My partner loves me so much that (s)he trusts our relationship to expand and be enriched by experiencing even more love from others.

New Core Belief #2

My relationship is so solid and trusting that we can experience other relationships freely. My partner is so satisfied with me and our relationship that having other partners will not threaten the bond we enjoy.

New Core Belief #3

There is an abundance of love in the world and there is plenty for everyone. Loving more than one person is a choice that can exponentially expand my potential for giving and receiving love.

The fact that these new beliefs sound so strange at first shows just how deeply the old paradigm beliefs about love and relationships are ingrained in our consciousness. It also underscores the importance of dissolving these old beliefs if we ever hope to enjoy multiple relationships without intense jealousy. You may choose to work on dislodging the old beliefs and incorporating these new beliefs on your own, with a partner, or in counseling.

Jealousy is almost always most intense right when one partner starts a new relationship, and usually subsides over time. A new romance shakes up everything in your life, including your existing relationship. I use the analogy that adding a new relationship is a little bit like having a baby, in a couple of important ways: while it can bring great joy and excitement to your lives, you are adding a new person to your life, and this creates a whole new dynamic in your relationship. Just like a new baby, a new relationship will change your schedule, your lifestyle, and take a lot of your time and energy, as well as adding a major source of stress to your life. And, like a new baby, it is an unknown quantity, and it is impossible to predict how it will change your life experience and what kind of intense feelings it will trigger. And flexibility and willingness to open yourself up to a completely new experience are crucial in adjusting to a new relationship.

At the beginning of a new relationship, fear of loss and abandonment are at their peak. Fear of the unknown and fear of change can be extremely uncomfortable as well, because, as one woman put it, "There's just no telling where this thing will go from here." As the drama of a new romance gradually settles into a more manageable relationship with clear parameters, most people relax and realize that this is not going to be fatal to the initial relationship. If you are the partner initiating a new relationship, you can significantly reduce your partner's initial jealousy through clear communication and reassurance that you are fully committed to staying with him or her and making every effort to meet your partner's needs.

The power imbalances caused by a new relationship can also aggravate jealousy. Particularly in a triad situation, where one person has two lovers and the other two only have one, an unfortunate dynamic of competition and a struggle for control can arise. This struggle can be minimized by encouraging all parties to communicate their needs openly, and by negotiating reasonable agreements that are fair to everyone. The person with two lovers should bend over backwards to avoid a power struggle and make sure both of his or her partners get enough time, attention, affection, commitment, and sex.

If someone in this position abuses power, they should be called on it immediately. Both lovers should become allies to demand a change in their partner's behavior, rather than allowing themselves to be manipulated against each other. Unless everyone cooperates and is careful of each other's feelings and needs, it is easy for one person to feel like the "odd person out." No one should feel powerless in a relationship — there is enough love for everyone to be satisfied.

8 Two Approaches for Managing Jealousy

There are two basic approaches for managing jealousy, which I call the *engineering model* and the *phobia model*.

The engineering model is an attempt to identify what situations and behaviors trigger your jealousy and to try to "engineer" those triggers out of your life by making rules to avoid that specific situation. The phobia model attempts to gradually expose yourself to things that trigger your jealousy, to take the emotional charge out of the situation with repeated experience.

Some successful examples of the engineering model:

George and Marsha lived together many years, but were on the verge of breaking up because of George's secondary relationship with Barbara. After a few counseling sessions, Marsha realized that she got much more jealous when George saw Barbara on weekends. The new relationship upset her schedule and shook up her sense of security, and she felt insulted that George was giving away his "prime time" to someone else. Marsha demanded that George reserve weekends for her and see Barbara only on weeknights. As soon as she was guaranteed every weekend with George, her jealousy became much more manageable. After several months, she felt secure enough that she told George he could see Barbara one weekend night each week, and they negotiated a schedule that seemed equitable for everyone.

Bob and Peter are two gay men in a committed relationship. Bob wanted sex much more often, so Peter told him to go to the baths and have casual sexual relationships with other men. However, he became angry and withdrawn when Bob actually went out, and was even less inclined to want sex. In counseling he revealed that he was worried that Bob might have unsafe sex with other men and be exposed to HIV/AIDS or other sexually transmitted infections. They agreed to both be re-tested for HIV, and negotiated a clear agreement that they would use condoms in any sexual activity outside of their relationship. After that, Peter's jealousy subsided so much that he began asking Bob to tell him about his sexual adventures. This sharing brought them closer and sexually aroused them both, and as a result they began having sex more frequently.

Sara, a bisexual woman, was involved with Dave, a straight man. Dave got involved with Helen. Helen had never been in an open relationship before, and was very jealous of Sara, demanding that Dave leave his relationship for her. Sara understood Helen's jealousy, so she encouraged Dave to spend more time with Helen to help her feel more secure. Sara also called Helen to reassure her that she welcomed her and wanted to cooperate to make this work out for all three of them. After a few months Helen gradually became less jealous and stopped making such extreme demands for Dave's time and attention.

Beth and Mark had agreed to an open relationship, but Beth was very jealous when Mark told her that he wanted to start a relationship with Janet. Beth asked Mark and Janet to give her a month to get used to the idea before becoming sexually involved, and they agreed to wait. As Beth got to know Janet she decided that Mark had excellent taste in women, and she gave them the green light to have a sexual relationship. The first few nights Mark spent with Janet were very hard for Beth; she couldn't sleep and was very frightened about the future, but she waited it out and her jealousy faded. Because she felt she had some control over the situation and had a voice in how it unfolded, and because her partner complied with her requests, her jealousy was minimized.

Jessica believed in open marriage but she became extremely jealous when her husband John initiated a sexual relationship with Carol. In counseling, it became clear that Jessica had already felt lonely and neglected for years because John was obsessed with his work and didn't give her enough time and enough sex. Behind her jealousy we as feeling of scarcity and deprivation, and an unmet need for love. As soon as John started spending more quality time with her, their intimacy was greatly enhanced, and her jealousy subsided.

Kate and Peggy are two bisexual women involved in a long-term relationship. Peggy got very jealous when her lover started a relationship with a man. In counseling, Peggy realized that she felt insecure about Kate's commitment to her. Behind her jealousy was an overwhelming fear of loss and abandonment, and she feared that Kate would leave her for this new man. Kate reassured her that she was fully committed to their relationship, and Peggy was able to move beyond jealousy to acceptance of her partner's new lover.

Greg had many affairs outside his marriage, but when his wife got involved with an attractive younger man that she met at the gym, he became very jealous and threatened divorce. In counseling, he admitted that he was feeling old and unattractive and felt very threatened by his wife's new lover. She reassured Greg that she loved him and that she was still very sexually attracted to him. Behind Greg's jealousy was the fear that his wife would reject him sexually, as well as his own insecurities about aging and loss of his desirability as a partner.

Notes On the Phobia Model

In the phobia model, I encourage clients to learn to accept jealousy as a normal but exaggerated response to a stressful, emotionally charged change in their lives. If someone were afraid of heights, a therapist would pinpoint exactly what situations frighten that person, and then gradually try to make those situations safe enough to tolerate. They would expose someone with a fear of heights first to a few steps and then to a ladder, and then going up an escalator, and eventually even going to the top of a hill or mountain. By gradually experiencing the situation that triggers the phobia, and by incrementally escalating that exposure, a person can slowly get used to situations that were once terrifying and overcome their fears.

Similarly, in managing jealousy with the phobia model, I ask clients to pinpoint as specifically as possible exactly what is triggering jealousy for them.

For example:

Susan identified that what upset her most about her husband Bill's affair was that he spent the night with Rachel, and Susan felt lonely sleeping alone. Bill agreed to come home every night, as long as he could spend a few evenings each week with Rachel. After a month, Susan realized that she was no longer so jealous, and she agreed to let him spend one night a week with Rachel, with the caveat that if she got really jealous she could call and ask him to come home. After a few more months she decided that it was okay for Bill to spend two nights a week with Rachel, and she only got jealous when Bill forgot her birthday and made a date with Rachel for that night. Throughout this process, Rachel was willing to be very flexible to accommodate Susan's demands, as she understood that securing Susan's cooperation was essential to making this relationship work for everyone. And for Susan, what worked was an incremental approach of exposing herself to exactly the situations she feared the most, and gradually learning to tolerate and even embrace this new situation.

Jim and Joan are a married couple. Joan became involved with Ruth. Because Joan had never been involved with a woman before, Ruth feared that Joan would drop her and go back to her comfortable heterosexual life. Ruth demanded more time and commitment from Joan to prove her commitment, but Jim got very jealous when Joan started spending more time with Ruth. Faced with two jealous lovers, Joan eventually negotiated an agreement: Jean would spend a few nights a week with Ruth, but each night she would call home to check in with Jim, and would go home if he was feeling too lonely and jealous. Jim agreed that if this worked out, after six months Ruth could move into their home and Joan would divide her time between them. After six months, Jim was not ready to let Ruth move in, and he asked to extend this for another three months, and by then his jealousy had subsided to the point where he welcomed her into the household.

While it's great to negotiate a plan so everyone has the same understanding and expectations, it is crucial to be flexible and willing to wait for all partners to be ready to take the next step. If any partner feels coerced into moving too fast, the phobic "fight or flight" mentality will kick in, and sabotage the outcome.

Visualize Your Jealousy Triggers

Using visualization and guided imagery often helps get down to the "nitty gritty" of what is causing jealousy. Close your eyes and visualize your partner initiating a new relationship with someone else, either someone they are currently interested in our involved with or with an imaginary "hypothetical lover." Watch the entire scenario unfold as if you were watching a film of the entire process.

Begin with when they first meet, the initial spark of interest, going on a date, having dinner or going out, going home with the new person, getting undressed, having sex, sleeping together, waking up in the morning, your lover coming back to you and telling you about the relationship, how your lover treats you, what it's like being with your lover again, etc. As if you had a remote control, press the pause button for a few moments at any point along the way where you feel discomfort or jealousy. Try to identify exactly what mix of emotions you are actually feeling at different points as the scenario unfolds.

Most people are surprised to find that visualizing their partner having another relationship like this is generally painless except at certain key moments; those "triggers" are different for each person. For instance, one woman discovered that going through the entire sequence was actually pleasurable except that she freaked out at visualizing her husband getting into "their" bed with another woman. She then made an agreement with him that he would only sleep with other women outside their home, either at the woman's house or at a hotel, and this made her feel safer. Another man found he was comfortable visualizing his partner having intercourse with another man, but became enraged when he visualized her having oral sex with the man. He considered fellatio as extremely intimate experience and asked her not to do that with any other man, and she agreed to that condition.

Another woman found the entire visualization pretty neutral, until she got to the part where after having sex, her husband talked to the new woman about his feelings for her. She realized that she didn't mind her partner having sex with another woman, but felt extremely threatened by him having an intimate conversation with her.

When you discover exactly what triggers your jealousy, it puts things in perspective. Realizing that you are only jealous of one or two pieces of the overall picture makes it much more manageable. After identifying your jealousy triggers, you have two basic choices. You can "engineer the problem away" by making agreements with your partner to avoid that particular behavior or situation, as shown in several previous examples. Or you can use the "phobia model," taking the risk of gradually exposing yourself to situations that provoke your jealousy, in the hopes that you will learn to tolerate and eventually feel comfortable with it.

It is important to keep in mind that there is no simple and easy solution to jealousy. It usually requires trial and error to discover what works for your individual situation. And jealousy can bring up many powerful feelings and unpredictable emotions. So be gentle with yourself and your partners, and don't expect instant changes. Try to be understanding of each person's needs and feelings. Make every effort to create a "win-win" situation for everyone by giving each person as much voice as possible in decisions and rule-making. And be willing to compromise to make sure everyone's needs are met.

Most people find that they need more rules and guidelines at first, to feel safer, have more predictability, and have fewer painful stimuli to manage. However, over time, most people discover that they can cope with more flexibility and fewer rules, because they feel more trusting of their partner's ability and commitment to handle things well, and they have seen through experience that their partner hasn't abandoned them. As people get more experience with other relationships, they develop a better skill set and are less likely to make mistakes which hurt their partner(s) and undermine trust.

What to Do If Your Partner Is Jealous

So what if your partner is the person experiencing jealousy? Sometimes dealing with a jealous lover is even more difficult than managing your own jealousy. When faced with a jealous partner, the most effective response is empathy and good communication. If you have made an effort to learn and implement some of the communication techniques laid out in Chapters 3 and 4, you will be well-equipped to be an ally to your partner in helping them cope with their feelings and work to resolve the jealousy.

First and foremost, listen carefully to your partner's words, non-verbal communication, and actions. Try to help them articulate exactly what they are feeling. Start by asking them if they are feeling more fear, sadness, or anger, and roughly the ratio of those three primary emotions. See if they can break it down further by describing in more detail what the feelings are and what they believe is the source of the source of these feelings. Acknowledge that you have heard and understood what your partner is experiencing. Even if you do not agree with their response and feel they are overreacting, you can understand that they are in pain and can see how they got there. Giving your partner that validation can go a long way toward reducing the jealousy and repair the intimacy that has been disrupted by this incident.

Don't try to "fix it" for them by trying to make those feelings go away or challenging the rational basis for those feelings. Allow them to have their feelings, and don't trivialize their pain or tell them they shouldn't feel that way.

See if you or your partner can identify what part you played in triggering the jealous response, and take responsibility for any of your own behaviors or attitudes that you could consider modifying to prevent creating jealousy in the future. You are bound to feel defensive, and your natural response will be to argue with your partner and justify your behavior. Resist that temptation, as no good will come of it! Instead, apologize for any actual mistakes you have made, even if your partner's response to those errors seems out of proportion to the situation. Ask your partner if they are willing to listen to your feelings about what happened. This step is important, as they may be feeling too wounded right now to hear how you experienced this, and you may have to agree to talk about your feelings later when they are feeling more resourceful and emotionally resilient.

Think carefully before making any agreements about what to do differently in the future. Don't agree to something just to appease your partner if you are going to resent it later, especially if you suspect that you will not keep this agreement. It is important to be willing to work together and compromise to enhance your partner's emotional safety, but don't be bullied by your partner's anger or fear. You will just create more distrust and jealousy in the future if you commit to something you know won't work for you, just because you feel manipulated or are so distressed by your partner's pain that you will do anything to alleviate it.

When your partner is in the midst of a jealousy attack, they need compassion and reassurance that they are loved. Things sometimes go from bad to worse, because their jealousy causes them to become so distraught that it triggers a defensive response and a huge argument. This is the worst possible reaction, because jealousy is about feelings and an argument is usually about intellectual analysis – you and your partner will be working at cross purposes and not actually communicating at all.

If you find yourself going down this path, ask for a brief time-out and take a few deep breaths. Then start over by trying to be present, hear your partner's feelings, and make your best effort to understand their experience and give them love and acceptance.

The Cost/Benefit Analysis of Jealousy

Despite their best efforts, some people find that the fear and pain evoked by an open relationship are too overwhelming. They may decide that it's just not worth the trouble, and may opt to return to a monogamous lifestyle. Or they may decide to take their time and work on their relationship to establish a stronger foundation of trust and security, while doing their individual personal growth work to understand and manage their jealousy.

Being involved in polyamorous relationships requires being willing to stretch ourselves and to tolerate a certain amount of discomfort, risk-taking, and uncertainty, especially at the beginning. While jealousy can be paralyzing at the outset, usually the balance of pain to pleasure will gradually shift until the enhanced satisfaction and joy will far outweigh the anxieties and pain. If you find that you and your partner(s) are unable to resolve jealous feelings on your own, get some outside help. Having a long talk with supportive friends can give you a fresh perspective and some honest feedback. Joining a support group can also be helpful, as other people who have been in similar situations may have good ideas for creative problem-solving. Individual counseling, couples counseling, or counseling for everyone involved in the situation can also create a safe environment for each person to express painful feelings and identify possible solutions.

Usually the first several months of exploring this new relationship style is the most difficult. If you have survived that and gotten your jealousy reasonably under control, congratulations! Now you are ready to learn about the other challenges experienced by polyamorous people.

Next Steps

Now that you have read Part Three and have developed the basic skill set necessary for creating open relationships, you are ready to learn how to sustain those relationships over time. Part Four describes some of the most common problems encountered in open relationships and provides advice on how to enhance the long-term success of your relationships.

LOVE IN ABUNDANCE

PART FOUR
Surviving And Thriving
In Open Relationships

9 Regulating Intimacy and Autonomy in Open Relationships

In any relationship, there will be some conflict over the regulation of intimacy and autonomy. However, this issue manifests with a different set of problems in polyamorous relationships than in monogamous couples.

No two people are perfectly matched in their needs for closeness and their need for separateness and privacy. This range extends from complete independence on one end of the spectrum to 24/7 "joined at the hip" coupledom at the other end. Each person has an ideal comfort zone of how much personal privacy, autonomy, and control over their own life they need, and how much love, intimacy, togetherness, and merging they want with a partner. One person in any given couple will always want more independence and more of a life of their own, and the other will always want more integration of their lives.

I find it useful to visualize a scale of zero to ten. Someone who is happiest at the zero end of the scale wants complete freedom and wants as much control as possible over every aspect of their life, and wants only a small amount of time and connection with a partner or partners. Someone at the ten end of the scale wants to merge as completely as possible with a partner or partners, and to spend all their time together, focusing all their attention on relationships.

Anyone who is below a two is probably not in a relationship, because they want more control, privacy, and independence than most relationships can tolerate. Such people are not comfortable giving enough time, attention, and intimacy to keep partners satisfied, so their relationships are unlikely to survive unless they are very casual relationships. People who are above an eight are also unlikely to be in a relationship, because they want more togetherness and merging than most people can tolerate, and their demands for time, attention, and loyalty would make most people feel smothered. Anyone between a two and an eight can find partners who want a similar balance between having a life of their own and being in a committed relationship. The key is to pick partners who are compatible, and relatively close to your number on the autonomy/intimacy scale.

For monogamous couples, discrepancies in these needs often prove fatal, because they are not allowed to meet their needs for love and intimacy outside of their primary relationship. If Partner A is a two on the scale and Partner B is an eight, they will be forever locked in a power struggle. Partner A will fight to the death to maintain some independence and control over as many aspects of their life as possible, carving out private time and space away from their partner. Partner B will experience a chronic scarcity of time, attention, affection, and closeness, and will lobby tirelessly for as much integration of their lives as possible, complaining bitterly and frequently of feeling neglected and unloved.

Each partner misinterprets the meaning of the other's needs and behaviors. Partner A believes that Partner B's demands for time and attention indicate that their partner is too controlling, demanding, and dependent. The phrases I hear most often are, "Why is she so needy and possessive?" "He must be so insecure and jealous to be constantly making all these demands." "I feel suffocated and I just want to run away." Partner B, on the other hand, believes that Partner A's need to distance represents a lack of caring, interest, and commitment, or an inability to tolerate intimacy. Some of the most common responses I hear are:

- "He doesn't really love me: if he loved me he would want to spend all his free time with me."

- "She's rejecting me: if she really cared about me she wouldn't go out with her friends."

- "He's afraid of intimacy; he just doesn't want to be close to me."

Usually, none of these "meanings" are accurate. Most people who are at the higher end of the scale are generally not clingy and insecure, they simply want and need a higher degree of connection, intimacy, and togetherness to feel loved and satiated. As one woman said to her partner, "I don't want to control you; I just want to know you and connect with you." Those who are at the lower end of the scale are usually not withdrawn, uncaring, or averse to intimacy or closeness with their partners. They simply need more time and space alone and more independence in order to maintain their own identity and feel safely differentiated from their partner. As the song says, "How can I miss you if you won't go away?"

Monogamous couples have few avenues for resolving these discrepancies. Often they break up because Partner A flees, due to the constantly escalating demands for intimacy, or Partner B can't stand feeling starved for love and affection and ends the relationship. Or else these incompatibilities lead to "cheating" and affairs, as Partner B realizes that they cannot get any additional attention from Partner A, so in desperation goes outside the relationship despite the monogamous agreement. Therapists used to call this kind of outside relationship a "marriage maintenance affair," as one partner is starting an outside relationship in order to get something they need which is too scarce in their primary relationship: intimacy, companionship, and emotional connection. The affair "maintains" the relationship, as Partner B is able to tolerate staying because their needs are being met elsewhere. Some people try to solve this dilemma by seeking emotional intimacy and connection from close friends or family members, but often the "missing ingredients" are affection, romance, and sex, which are off-limits for monogamous people outside the primary relationship.

Polyamorous people are at a distinct advantage over monogamous couples in this regard; open relationships can solve some of the problems created by different autonomy/intimacy needs. If a discrepancy exists, any partner can seek other partners to meet their needs. In addition, if a partner is feeling smothered or overwhelmed by their partner's demands for intimacy, they can encourage their partner to seek outside partners to take the pressure off them and lessen conflicts over their incompatible needs.However, this can lead to some interesting new problems.

For example:

Miriam was an eight on the scale, and her husband Saul was a three. Miriam spent years feeling lonely, rejected, and unloved because Saul, a biochemist, spent a lot of weekends working on research in his lab, and when at home he wanted to spend a lot of time surfing the Internet, reading scientific articles, and watching movies. Because they had agreed on an open relationship, Miriam became involved in two secondary relationships with other men. One of the new partners was a five on the scale and the other was a six, so both were much better matched with her in their needs. She began spending a lot of time on these two intense new romances. She was delighted that they each pursued closeness with her and wanted a lot of her time and attention. Because her needs were beginning to be satiated, she started to feel more like a five or six on the scale. Before long the demands of her two new lovers became so time- and energy-consuming that her primary partner began to complain of being neglected, and she began to feel overwhelmed by all the pressure of meeting the needs of all three partners. Eventually she felt compelled to cut back on her outside relationships, and one of her lovers left her because he felt he was not getting enough time and attention.

This example illustrates a phenomenon I have seen frequently with poly couples: someone starting at one number on the scale and moving up or down depending on their relationship situation. Conversely, couples often become polarized when their needs diverge. For instance, one couple I worked with started out with one person at a four and the other at a six, but after fighting about it for years they found themselves much farther apart at a two and a seven. Because they both felt so pressured by the other's needs and demands, they each became more rigid and dug their heels in, refusing to compromise and unable to find common ground. Such behavior creates a power struggle that is difficult to resolve.

Often, differing needs regarding intimacy and autonomy are the key impetus for couples to become polyamorous. However, this difference can sometimes sow the seeds of the demise of the primary relationship. This often happens to couples who are not truly polyamorous people but are only trying an open relationship as a conflict resolution strategy. The danger is that the partner who goes outside the relationship for intimacy is likely to choose someone who is more closely matched with their intimacy needs, and may decide to leave the primary relationship for a monogamous relationship with the new partner. Couples who are considering polyamory as a solution to discrepancies in their needs for intimacy and autonomy should think carefully about whether this could potentially jeopardize their relationship. Take a brutally honest look about whether in fact you actually want a monogamous relationship but are simply incompatible with this particular partner.

A more difficult problem can be created if the person who is at the lower end of the intimacy/autonomy scale chooses to enter into outside relationships.

For example:

John is a two and Alice is an eight. Alice is generally pretty satisfied because she has been having numerous outside relationships to supplement her intimacy needs that cannot be accommodated within the primary relationship. John is happy that Alice is no longer pressuring him for more time, intimacy, and attention. Then, John decides he also would like to try having an outside relationship, or (more often) someone else makes a pass at him and he decides to go for it. Alice panics about this new development, and everyone around them is puzzled. Much talk ensues about "What's good for the goose is good for the gander," and "You can dish it out but you can't take it," and other such proclamations of a double standard of behavior in which Alice wants to have the freedom to pursue outside relationships but is unhappy when John does likewise. While on the surface Alice looks like a hypocrite, in fact, her behavior makes perfect sense. She has been living with scarcity for the entire duration of the relationship. Alice has only managed to live with what she considers the "bare minimum" because she has been outsourcing her surplus needs for intimacy to other partners. She knows from years of painful personal experience that John has a low tolerance for intense intimacy and has a finite amount of time and energy to devote to relationships. As a result, she suspects that if he begins to devote some of that to another partner there is a strong likelihood that she will receive even less than she has been getting so far, which has been sub-optimal. So she wants him to abandon the other

relationship and reserve his relationship energy for her. While it may seem unfair that she is reluctant to support his polyamourous behavior, her fears are grounded in reality, from seeing first-hand that he has a particular set of needs around intimacy, autonomy, and privacy, and that those needs are likely to prove incompatible with sustaining two relationships.

There is no perfect solution for this dilemma. Often someone like John can only discover what his limits are by trying to maintain two relationships and finding out the hard way what amount of intimate connection he can tolerate. Sometimes the story has a happy ending because John learns to stretch himself and get more comfortable devoting more time and space to relationships. Or he finds he cannot manage two serious relationships and instead pursues only casual sex partners or one-time play partners. Or he is able to compartmentalize outside relationships by having a long-distance relationship with someone out of town who he can stay in touch with by phone and email but only see once in a while. Often, someone like John will have an intense love affair that will take up a lot of time and energy but end rather soon and lead to him saying something like, "That was really amazing and wonderful but I don't think I'll ever do that again! It was just too exhausting and stressful and I 'm kind of glad life is back to normal." Sometimes, however, the ending is not so happy, as John goes merrily forward in pursuing an intense relationship and is unable to give enough time and attention to his primary partner. Since she is already feeling chronically deprived, if the amount of romantic love and attention then drops below that marginally satisfying minimum amount, it often doesn't take long for her to feel completely starved and end the relationship.

I encourage anyone who is in an open relationship to think carefully about where you are on the autonomy/intimacy scale, and consider how that may affect your relationships. How much time and energy can you reliably devote to intimate relationships, how much intimacy and connection do you reliably need, and how much privacy and independence do you need on a regular basis for your life to feel satisfying and balanced? Look back into your relationship history to identify patterns in how this issue has affected you.

In past relationships, were you often feeling a need for more closeness and feeling frustrated and lonely because you did not get enough time and attention from your partner? If so, you are probably a 6, 7, or 8 on the scale. You would probably be wise to make sure you seek partners who are also a 5 or above on the scale, and are likely to want a similar amount of attention and connection. However, you can get in a lot of trouble by picking two or more partners who, like yourself, are "high maintenance." For instance, if you are an 8 and you pick two partners who are both 8s, you will be besieged by an intense demand for your time and attention, and it is unlikely that you will be able to deliver enough time, attention, and intimacy to keep both partners happy. If you do the math, it will be obvious that no one person can have enough energy or time to satisfy two partners who need a very high degree of connection, and their demands will eventually lead to the collapse of at least one of these relationships.

A good rule of thumb for poly people is to pick at least one partner who is a few numbers lower than you are on the scale. For instance, it works well for an 8 to pick a 7 or 8 as a primary partner as long as any additional partners are around 5 or 6. This configuration works because you can reserve enough time and energy for your primary partner and still have some left over for an additional partner who is around a 5 or 6 and able to be satisfied with less attention.

On the other hand, in past relationships, were you usually the person trying to set boundaries to keep your partners from taking up too much space in your life and getting too much control over your time and attention? If so, you are probably a 2, 3, or 4 on the scale. You are probably smart to pick a primary partner who is also around a 2, 3, or 4 and who highly values their independence and wants to have a lot of separate time and a life of their own separate from the couple experience. However, as mentioned above, it is wise to pick at least one partner that is a few numbers lower on the scale than you are, as otherwise you will experience too much demand from multiple partners for time and attention and you will be overwhelmed and smothered, or will get trapped in power struggles with your partners because they want more intimacy and connection than you can reliably deliver.

A frequently seen configuration is for someone who is a 2, 3, or 4 to pick a 2, 3, or 4 as a primary and pick a 2 as a secondary, so they can consistently provide enough time and romantic attention to keep both partners satisfied and not create a deficit. Some people who are at a 2 or 3 find that it works best to limit their outside relationships to very casual play partners, to go to sex parties with the primary partner, to have one-time sexual partners, or some other "low-maintenance" outside relationships that do not exhaust their tolerance for intimacy and socializing and do not take too much time away from the primary relationship. Some people who are at the lower end of the scale at a 2 or 3 decide they do not want to have primary relationships at all, and do better having two or more non-primary relationships where there is not such a big demand on them for intimacy and togetherness. For some people this is the ideal lifestyle and satisfies their needs for romance, sex, love, and companionship without the pressures of constant interaction and intimacy.

I often suggest a brief exercise to couples which may be useful to you in your relationships. Take a piece of paper and first write down on the left side of the paper where you think you are on the intimacy/autonomy scale. Then on the right side of the paper, write down the number that you think best represents where you partner is on the scale. Then compare notes with your partner and see whether either of you guessed right about the other's number. Have a brief discussion with your partner about what problems this has caused in your relationship and talk about how you might be able to support each other in meeting your needs for both intimacy and autonomy. Try to avoid jumping to conclusions about what your partner's feelings "mean," and try to avoid judging your partner's needs and desires for more or less connection or for more or less independence. Remember that each person has their own unique needs, and focus on ways to compromise and to come up with solutions to meet each partner's needs.

Now that you have an understanding of how your needs for intimacy and autonomy can impact your relationships, the next chapter will address some of the ways in which these needs can lead to difficulties.

Are You In Poly Hell?: Common Pitfalls In Open Relationships

Many people who are in a primary relationship stumble into an outside relationship either by choice or by chance. This event can end beautifully or terribly, depending on the skills and motivations of all the individuals involved. Here are some of the most common problems that develop in this situation, and some ideas for either avoiding them or effectively addressing them should they arise.

New Relationship Energy

The most typical poly dilemmas are take place when one partner devotes too much time and energy to an outside relationship and to some extent ignores or neglects the partner at home.

On the one hand, this is understandable. A new romance, even if casual or "secondary," is often imbued with that infamous "New Relationship Energy," or NRE, which involves a lot of fantasy and projection. When we first get involved with someone, we don't know them very well yet and do not know all their bad habits and annoying behaviors, so it's easy to imagine them to be the perfect person and ideal romantic partner we have been longing for. There is an unbeatable combination of novelty, mystery, and chemistry, mixed with our own romantic fantasies and the fact that our new partner is on their best behavior and trying to impress us by exhibiting their most attractive qualities. So there is some excuse for getting distracted by the "shiny new toy" aspect of a hot new love affair, wanting to spend a lot of time exploring this new person, thinking about them obsessively.

In an open relationship, the existing primary relationship most often involves living together and sharing chores, bills, kids, and all the stresses of everyday life. It is tough for that long-term couple relationship to deliver the intensity and excitement of a new, responsibility-free relationship. Ironically, part of the problem is that the new relationship makes you realize that your primary relationship is not quite as hot and wild as it was in the beginning, and that contrast creates nostalgia and longing for the mad passion you once experienced.

On the other hand, it is understandable that the partner who is left at home will feel extremely hurt and threatened by this new relationship that seems to be taking over your life. So some compromise must be struck between the compelling desire to bask in this fun and exciting new experience and the primary partner's need for reassurance, security, and attention.

The most common problems growing out of this tension between competing needs are what I call demotion, displacement, and intrusion. I will discuss each of these problems briefly.

Demotion

The primary partner has previously had you all to him- or herself, and has not had to share your time, affection, attention, and loyalty with another lover. Most partners take this hegemony for granted without thinking about it explicitly. When a new partner enters the picture, suddenly the primary partner feels demoted from "the one and only" to being one of two partners. This is a huge shock, and often very distressing to anyone who is experiencing it for the first time. Most of us have no particular training for sharing our lover's romantic attention with someone else, and many people find it so disorienting and painful that they describe it in words like these: "I felt like I had been kicked in the stomach" or "I suddenly felt I didn't know what my place was any more or what my status was in my partner's life."

Some amount of demotion is inevitable. Some portion of the partner's attention will necessarily be diverted from the primary relationship to the new partner. Everyone has to face the undeniable reality that things are different now: they can no longer depend on having a monopoly on their partner's romantic energy. It doesn't mean their partner loves them less or that they are less important to their partner, it just means that another person has some small claim on their partner's time and affection.

Making this adjustment is usually painful and takes time. This transition can be eased by clear and loving communication about how this change will affect the primary relationship. Both people need to articulate their needs and negotiate what the partners can reasonably expect from each other. How much time will your partner be spending with this new person? What kind of boundaries will bracket that relationship? What types of activities are allowed in this new relationship? Will some things be off-limits and reserved for the primary relationship? The partner who has initiated an outside relationship can reduce their partner's anxiety and jealousy through consistent reassurance of their commitment to the relationship, and by consistently keeping agreements in order to foster greater trust.

During this initial transition, the partner who is feeling "demoted" often reports experiencing sadness, betrayal, distrust, a sense of loss and grieving, and fear of abandonment. The other partner often makes the situation worse by denying that there is any loss, ridiculing or dismissing their partner's fears, and stressing that this new development will enhance the primary relationship. While this denial may be sincere, and is intended to reassure the partner that they have nothing to fear and that the primary relationship is not in jeopardy, it is bound to backfire by making the partner feel invalidated. Instead, it is important to acknowledge that their partner *has* lost something: they have lost the primacy of being the one and only lover, and they need to grieve that loss even though in the long run the new relationship may have an overall positive effect on the primary relationship.

Some people have such intense reactions to this change that one suspects there may be some past trauma that is being triggered or old wounds re-opened.

For example:

Mel thought he would be fine with his wife Susan having outside partners. However, when Susan did become romantically involved with another man, he had panic attacks and episodes of rage. He eventually realized the source of this reaction. For him, this situation was very reminiscent of his childhood, as he was an only child until he was ten years old, when his parents had another child. He experienced intense sibling rivalry with his baby brother as he felt betrayed by his parents for demoting him from the "one and only" to one of two sons. With the birth of a sibling, things will never be the same again, as the children will always have to share their parents' love, loyalty, time, and attention. This change entails loss and grief, even if eventually the joy of having a sibling may outweigh the loss of the parents' total devotion. Susan's outside romantic involvement caused Mel to re-experience his old feelings of loss and abandonment.

Betty experienced intense episodes of jealousy and felt completely betrayed when her primary partner Anita became involved with another woman. In counseling it emerged that she had been raised by a single mother and had her undivided love and attention. Her mother married a new man when she was nine years old. Betty was devastated that a big portion of her mother's love and attention was now being diverted to the husband, and she felt ignored and left out. The new poly situation was bringing back those same feelings of shock, betrayal and exclusion. Betty needed to work through those feelings and realize that she was no longer a helpless child; as an adult, she could take care of herself and ask for what she needed to feel safe.

Cheryl had a similarly intense reaction of fear and emotional paralysis when her husband Dean started a relationship with another woman. She realized that she was projecting the past onto this situation, as her previous husband had started a secret affair and left her for another woman. Once she received reassurance that Dean was committed to their marriage and was not going to leave her, her fears subsided.

For those of us who find that our reactions are more extreme than seem warranted, counseling or a support group may help you discover the origin of these feelings and learn to separate past trauma from the present poly situation.

Displacement

Displacement refers to the experience of feeling that a partner's outside relationship is beginning to receive so much time, attention, and loyalty that it is crowding out the primary relationship. Often the partner exacerbates the situation by spending too much time seeing the new partner, calling or emailing the new partner, making lots of romantic gestures like cards, gifts, and affection, while ignoring the primary partner's need for romantic attention. People who are trying out an open relationship for the first time often make this mistake, which can be chalked up to a learning experience. Unfortunately, however, some people repeat this mistake again and again with subsequent partners.

Because the outside relationship is new, unpredictable, tenuous, and mysterious, there is a tendency to become infatuated and pursue the new partner intensely. Since the primary relationship is stable, secure, and familiar, it is often taken for granted while the new relationship gets more of the romantic attention. The partner at home feels abandoned, unloved, and disrespected, and begins to feel that they are being displaced by the new person.

Some feelings of displacement are almost inevitable. However, they can be minimized if the partner with the outside relationship is diligent in providing adequate time, attention, and loving gestures to the primary partner as well as the new partner. Spending quality time together and having special dates, as well as giving romantic attention to the primary partner, can go a long way towards reassuring them of love, commitment, and intention to sustain the relationship.

Some people have expressed confusion about the difference between demotion and displacement, and in fact they are similar. However, demotion is about the change in status of the primary relationship, as the partner no longer has an exclusive relationship and no longer has the same rights and roles as before. Displacement is more about the loss of time, loyalty, and attention, and having to learn to share aspects of their partner with another. So demotion is about loss of status and roles. Displacement is more about logistics and the practical reality of less time and attention from your partner.

Intrusion

This word refers to the way an outside relationship has the tendency to invade the time and space of the primary relationship and make the primary partner feels unsafe in the relationship. Often the person having the new relationship is under the influence of lust and infatuation, and feels so motivated to pursue this exciting new love affair that they ignore their primary partner's pleas for time and attention. They rationalize that they must focus on the new partner to solidify that relationship or it may not survive. At the same time, they see the primary relationship as stable and secure. As a result, they take their relationship for granted and fail to grasp that it needs maintenance and sustenance in order to thrive. When we are spending time with our primary partner, we may feel the need or desire to stay in close contact with the other partners, and may spend a little or a lot of time phoning, texting, emailing them, or chatting with them on-line, when we are "supposed" to be giving our attention to the primary partner at that moment. This can be very painful for the present partner, whether we do this openly in front of them, or excuse ourselves and leave the room, or do it while they are in the shower or napping.

Intrusion can be especially difficult to manage at the beginning of a new relationship, when passion and infatuation are high, and there is often excess drama that feels compelling to resolve. At the same time the primary partner's anxieties and jealousy is likely to be higher at the beginning of a new relationship and they are likely to be even more sensitive to the other partner invading their time and space.

Other relationships can also intrude in less obvious ways, such as one partner being too tired for sex after staying out late the night before with the other partner, or being distant and distracted during a date because of some intense drama going on in the new relationship. We may make the mistake of talking way too much about the new relationship, letting discussions about that relationship take over the time we spend with our primary partner.

Scheduling conflicts and logistics can also feel very invasive to the primary relationship. Now that there is a new person in the picture, schedules need to be renegotiated to include dates with both partners, and special occasions like birthdays, holidays, and anniversaries need to be taken into consideration. How will the new relationship affect vacation and travel plans? Will there be a reluctance to take trips because the new partner will be left alone? Is it okay to take a weekend trip or longer vacation with the new partner? All these possibilities can make the primary partner feel unsafe, as if their world is no longer secure and everything is up for grabs, and make the situation even more painful.

The damage done by neglect during this phase often proves fatal to the primary relationship, because the primary partner is experiencing a scarcity of time and romance with their partner, and their pleas for their partner to focus attention on the relationship fall on deaf ears. As one man said, "Not only was she spending most of her time with this other guy, whenever I tried to tell her how I felt she ignored me and didn't seem to care that I was very unhappy." Eventually they may feel so abandoned and humiliated that they leave the relationship, because the cumulative effect of unmet needs necessitates them withdrawing their own relationship energy from the primary relationship. They will begin detaching in preparation for ending the relationship, or will divert their relationship focus to another partner (or partners) who will be more attentive and available.

Unfortunately, it is only at the point that the primary partner decides to end the relationship that the partner usually takes their demands seriously, because they have been oblivious, and naively believed that the relationship was secure. And by then it is usually too late to repair the damage, as their partner is already on their way out the door, and feels so mistreated and distrustful they are unlikely to be deterred.

Some amount of intrusion is inevitable in any open relationship, as it is impossible to neatly compartmentalize relationships so completely that no relationship will ever intrude in any way on another. It is likely that there will be times when one partner is in acute need, such as needing to be driven to the emergency room while you are in the middle of a date with the primary partner, or someone will be having a "poly meltdown" and needing to talk at a very inconvenient moment. There will also be likely to be a few "oops" moments in any poly relationship, such as accidentally scheduling a date with one partner on the other partner's birthday and having to humbly ask to reschedule. And there will also be moments when we are distracted by something going on in an outside relationship and may need to make contact with that partner while at home or on a date with our primary partner. These do not have to be catastrophic, and can be handled rationally and graciously by most partners as long as there is some valid reason for the intrusion and they don't happen too frequently.

Like most things about open relationships, these small intrusions usually become much easier to handle the longer the relationship goes on. This is especially true if we treat both our primary partner and outside partners lovingly and respectfully, listening carefully to their experiences and their feelings, and making a good faith effort to meet their needs and avoid pushing their buttons. Some of the charge goes out of the situation after a while as all partners prove to be reliable and trustworthy, and give each other more slack as time goes on.

I usually suggest that each person give each of their partners three "Get out of jail free" cards. What I mean by this is that you can just assume that their will be some intrusions that will cause pain, and that your partners will be likely to make a few mistakes on the learning curve in balancing their own needs and the needs of multiple partners. Each time some intrusion happens that creates great distress, they use up one of their "Get out of jail free" cards. Hopefully they will try their best to avoid hurting you, and it will take them a while to use up all three cards. By then it is likely that you will be much more accustomed to the situation and much more tolerant of occasional invasions into your relationship, and the partner will have a much better skill set to avoid repeating their mistakes.

In the meantime, it is important to establish some boundaries about how much, how often, and in what ways the outside relationship may intrude on the primary relationship. By the same token it is important to make agreements on how much the primary relationship can intrude on outside relationships, as those relationships deserve protection as well.

Some couples establish guidelines on whether it is okay for someone to phone, email, or text their other partners while in the presence of the primary partner. Some people decide it is fine to discreetly email the other partner while you are on your computer doing other things anyway. Some agree to text or phone their other partners while the present partner is occupied doing something else, such as on the phone with relatives or putting the kids to bed. Some agree that it is fine to leave the room and call or email a partner, as long as a specific time limit is kept, so that it does not drain too much time or connection away from the present partner or trigger abandonment fears. There is no right or wrong way to do this, as long as everyone is comfortable with the situation and can tolerate the degree of intrusion involved.

Many couples find it most difficult to manage the more subtle intrusions, such as talking too much about outside partners, or being tired or emotionally unavailable due to thinking about or spending too much time on outside relationships. Sometimes it helps to commit to more time together, even if it means taking time away from work or some other activity, to give the primary relationship more attention. Going to a poly support group or social group, where you can talk with others about what works for them and can see healthy models of working out these conflicts, can help. Often, couples counseling can help navigate these perilous situations and give both partners a "reality check" on reasonable expectations and standards of behavior.

If you are experiencing an intolerable degree of displacement, demotion, and/or intrusion in your relationship, you are in "poly hell," and need to intervene in order to change your partner's behavior and stabilize your relationship. Being in an open relationship does not mean being a doormat. You have a right to expect your partner to make every effort to remain physically and emotionally available to meet your needs for time, attention, affection, intimacy, and sex, despite outside relationships. Sometimes counseling is necessary to help turn things around if one partner is not responding to their partner's needs, or if one partner is making unreasonable or unrealistic demands.

The next chapter will discuss some of the options for managing your living arrangements. There are many possibilities for living with one or more partner in an open relationship, and there are many factors to consider in assessing which living style is best for you.

11 Poly Living Styles: Should We All Live Together?

Over the past twenty years that I have been counseling poly people professionally, I've noticed a strong belief that one form of polyamory is somehow superior to others. Over and over I hear from clients that "real" polyamory is a group marriage where three or more adult partners live together in one household, sharing finances, children, and housework as a family unit. When I ask people where they got that idea, they seem baffled, saying, "I just thought that's what polyamory is." Most of these clients are very unhappy because they have tried that model at least once (and often more times with different partners) and it crashed and burned after a few months or a year. They say they "feel like a failure" because they have aspired to live what they see as the ultimate poly ideal and have not been able to sustain it.

I have often wondered why the "living together as a family under the same roof" scenario seems firmly rooted in our community as the one true path of polyamory. It may be because it is similar to the nuclear family that many of us are accustomed to: it's just like being married except you're married to more than one person. It may also have become our popular mythology because this model has frequently appeared in science fiction books, such as Heinlein's portrayal of "line marriage" and other group marriage models. And past attempts at communal utopias like the Onieda Community and others have included group marriages, and this, too, may have encouraged us to see this as the "correct" form of polyamory.

Whatever its origin as a model, the majority of people who try this "all living together" model find that it does not work for them. The more you are informed about the challenges and potential pitfalls, the more accurately you can assess the viability of this model for you, and can take steps to maximize your chances for success.

I've seen literally hundreds of threesomes and foursomes move in together as poly families, and I can count on my fingers the ones who have been able to sustain their family for more than two years. For those who succeed, the rewards are manifold:

- multiple adults to share cooking, housework, and childcare,
- multiple incomes to achieve a more comfortable standard of living and provide long- term financial security,
- more economical and ecological living through pooling resources,
- plenty of companionship,
- stable romantic and sexual relationships, and
- a built-in social life and community.

The three key ingredients for making this model work are:

- an extremely high degree of compatibility among all partners on all aspects of living together,
- a high degree of flexibility and willingness to compromise and accommodate the needs of all family members, and
- excellent interpersonal skills, good communication, and healthy boundaries.

All three of these are important to any polyamorous relationship, but are absolute necessities if you are all living together.

Here are some examples of poly families that have succeeded at this very difficult task:

Jill, Andrew, and Jason are a poly family who have lived together for ten years. All three are bisexual. Jill and Andrew had been together two years when they got involved with Jason. Their apartments were too small, so they rented a bigger house where they each could have their own bedroom.

Most nights all three sleep together in a king-size bed, but they make frequent dates to spend intimate time separately with each partner. They spend most of their time together, cooking, gardening, meditating at a Buddhist center, and doing political work for peace. Outside sexual relationships are allowed as long as they do not become so consuming that they interfere with family life. Each contributes 50% of their income to the family checking account to pay for rent, food, and utilities, and each keeps the other half of their income for their own use.

Roberto, Jim, and Ed are a gay male triad that has lived together for twelve years. They identify as a BDSM family rather than calling themselves poly. Roberto is a dominant and both Jim and Ed are submissives. Jim is Roberto's husband and Ed is Roberto's boy. Roberto and Ed have jobs and support the family financially. Ed works full-time in their home cooking, cleaning, and gardening. All money is pooled in a single bank account, but Roberto makes all financial decisions. Occasionally, Roberto brings other men into the house for sex and BDSM activities with all three partners, but these relationships are casual.

Ann and Benjamin are a heterosexual couple who both identify as dominants in the BDSM community. Ann has another male partner, Allen, who lives with them and identifies himself as Ann's slave. Benjamin also has a female submissive, Jenna, who lives with them. Ann and Benjamin have been married for twenty years, and Allen and Jenna have lived with them about five years.

Angela, Carlos and Janine have been living together for six years as a poly family. Angela and Carlos were already living together when Angela got involved with Janine. Janine also expressed an interest in Carlos, so they became sexually involved, and eventually they bought a home and all moved in together. Angela travels about two weeks out of every month for her job, so Carlos spends private time with Janine when Angela is away. When she is in town, Angela divides her time equally between the two relationships. They each keep separate checking accounts and keep their finances separate. However, all three are co-owners in the house. Since Janine is a carpenter and does most of the repairs on the house, she pays less of the household expenses. They are polyfidelitous, so no sexual relationships are allowed outside the family.

Denise, Millie, and Joseph have lived together for seven years as a family. Millie and Joseph's two children also live with them. Denise was married to Bob, and the two couples met over the Internet and courted. Denise and Bob moved from LA to the Bay Area to move in with Joseph and Millie to form a poly family. However, many conflicts developed because Bob was unhappy with the behavior of the children, as well as disagreements over finances. Eventually Bob moved out and he and Denise divorced. Denise decided to continue living with Millie, Joseph, and their children. They are now seeking another man to join their family. Currently they pool all their incomes, as they are saving money to buy a bigger house, and Denise is trying to get pregnant. All three have jobs, but Millie identifies as the primary parent and works outside the home only two days a week to give her more time with the children.

As you can see, three seems to be the magic number. I have not personally seen any poly household with more than three partners that survived for more than a year. I've seen several households with a primary couple who add another couple and eventually end up as a threesome. It seems quite rare that all four people are compatible and flexible enough to handle the demands of a poly family, and eventually one of the four opts out. I've also seen some group marriages where two or even three of the partners stay together for many years but the fourth or fifth partners leave and are replaced by new people every year or so. It's certainly possible, however, that there are successful foursomes or moresomes out there.

Challenges of Living Together As a Poly Family

So why is this model so difficult to sustain? Ironically, the reasons most of these families disintegrate so quickly have nothing to do with polyamory. Instead, they fail because of the difficulties of living together:

conflicts over housework, kids, money, space, and privacy. Everyone must be able to reach agreement on all these questions:

- where to live
- what house or apartment to buy or rent
- whether or not to pool financial resources
- how much money to spend and what expenditures are acceptable
- how clean to keep the house and who will be responsible for which chores
- what kind of food to buy and who will cook meals
- how much privacy or personal time each partner will have
- how much time will be spent as a family
- whether to have children, how many children, how they will be cared for, and what styles of child-rearing are acceptable.

Most people find it difficult to connect with even one partner they can successfully live with for the long haul, much less two, three, or more. I've seen poly families fall apart over such seemingly small decisions as whether to buy a new car, what color to paint the house, what school to send the kids to, whether to allow meat in the house, or even "Who is leaving dirty dishes in the sink?"

Financial Issues and Power Struggles

Conflicts over finances are a common cause of poly divorces. One partner feels they are working harder than the others and contributing more to supporting the household, and pressures the others to make more money. Or one member wants to spend more money on travel or eating out or buying clothes, and other partners want to save money for retirement or spend it to put a new roof on the house or send the kids to private school.

Conflicts over money sometimes arise when one partner makes substantially more money than others and feels that because they contribute more financially they should have more say in family decisions. Or the higher wage earner feels that their financial contribution exempts them from doing any housework, and others don't necessarily agree.

Other conflicts center on how much responsibility the partners feel is appropriate to take on for each partner's extended family. One family broke up when one woman's thirty-year-old daughter and her two small kids moved in with them after a messy divorce. She expected her poly family to provide free rent, food, and childcare for her daughter and grandchildren, and the family balked at "supporting someone else's kids." Another family fell apart when one man's elderly father developed Alzheimer's. He wanted his father to move in and be financially supported and physically cared for by his poly family, but they did not feel this was their responsibility, and doing so would mean major sacrifices and a heavy workload. It's best to clarify how such possible situations will be handled before you move into together so there are no surprises. Think carefully about what you are willing to commit to, and whether you can in fact live up to that agreement.

Financial matters can get even more complicated when poly partners move into an existing home owned by one individual or couple. The homeowner(s) will almost certainly feel territorial about controlling the space and want more power over decisions in the family. If other members move in as renters, their partner(s) will also be their landlord, setting up an unfortunate power dynamic that can lead to messy financial, legal, and interpersonal problems. Even if the new members buy into the house as part owners, they will probably always feel like it is not really their home since the original owners were there first and have "seniority."

For example:

The Andersons, a heterosexual couple, met the Blythes, another heterosexual couple, and fell in love. The Blythes eventually agreed to sell their small house and move into the Andersons' larger home. The Blythes made a substantial down payment and became 50% owners in the Andersons' house. However, the Blythes couldn't move any of their furniture in because there "wasn't any room" (the Andersons were very attached to the current décor). Joan Anderson became distraught when Marta Blythe tried to cook in "her" kitchen, and found she wanted total control over food-buying and cooking. Bill Anderson had painted the whole house his favorite colors, and was dismayed when Tom Blythe wanted to paint the Blythes' bedroom a different color. The Blythes had to get rid of all their books because the Andersons' books took up all the space in all the many bookcases in every room in the house. As you can guess, this poly marriage did not last.

In my experience, it often works better for everyone in a poly family to move into a new, neutral space that no one is already emotionally attached to. That way everyone is starting off fresh with the same amount of power and investment in creating a home that works for everyone.

Struggles Over Household Tasks

In disagreements over housework and cooking, battle lines are also often drawn between genders, with the women complaining that the men expect the women to cook and clean up after them. (Of course, women can be slobs, too, or can drive other partners crazy with clutter.) I've seen numerous poly families wrecked because of conflicts between one person who is a neat freak and another who is very sloppy. It's bound to escalate as the person who likes the house clean will become so resentful they will eventually move out or try to evict the sloppy partner. Some households have tried to solve this by hiring a professional cleaning service to keep the house clean, but many can't afford this or believe strongly that everybody should clean up their own mess. Some families agree to support one member of the family financially so that person can stay home and be responsible for most of the housework, cooking, and childcare.

Cooking can also be a "black hole" in poly households – either no one has time to cook, or one person feels they are doing way more than their share. And many households have great difficulty reaching consensus on what foods to buy and cook. Some members want all organic foods or a vegan diet, some won't drink coffee or alcohol, others will eat cheese and eggs but no meat, some eat fish, some are allergic to wheat. One member may abhor all processed foods, while another can't live without pizza and ice cream. Some try to solve this by only buying and serving the foods that everyone can agree on. This way, individuals can buy a few of their own favorite foods for themselves out of their own money, but they won't be included in shared meals.

Conflicts Over Children and Child-Rearing

Yet another issue that has doomed many poly families is incompatibility around children and child-rearing. Many poly families are "blended" families, with one or more children from previous relationships. This blending often creates conflicts over scheduling custody arrangements with ex-spouses, as well as complex child-care assignments for family members. Some family members do not want to care for other members' children. Sometimes the biological parent(s) object strongly to other partners providing limits or discipline for their children. There can be sharp disagreements among multiple partners over children's behavior, bedtimes, homework, activities, diet, etc, and it can be impossible to reach consensus. Disputes over child care sometimes break down along gender lines: the women in the household are doing way more than their share of the parenting and want the men to pull their weight. I know one poly family where the women left the family and took the children with them because they felt so unsupported by their male partners in child-rearing duties.

If there are not children when the poly family initially is formed, "irreconcilable differences" may develop if one partner wants children and the others don't. I've seen several poly families disband because one partner could not persuade the others to agree to having children. Another family split up because one couple already had children and the other woman in the triad wanted to have a child, but the couple didn't want to raise any more children.

Differing Expectations About Privacy and Togetherness

Disagreements about "privacy versus togetherness" derail many poly families. Living together makes it more challenging for each member and each relationship to have privacy and personal autonomy. Relationships that previously were private suddenly become part of family life.

Many families founder when trying to strike a balance between the needs of each person, each relationship, and the family as a whole. The regulation of intimacy and autonomy, as discussed in Chapter 9, can be just as challenging between family members as within a couple.

For example, how much time are you allowed to have to yourself, to just shut the door of your room and read a book? Are all partners expected to be home for dinner every night, or can you go out with your friends instead? If you want private time with one partner to cuddle or go to a movie, is that okay, or are you expected to include the other partners? Does each partner have their own room, or are you expected to share your personal space? Do you devise a schedule for which partner to sleep with on which nights or the week, or is it based on how you each feel each day, or will you all sleep together in one room? Many families discover that each partner has very different expectations about the amount of personal freedom and privacy, and how much control the family will exert over their time and activities. It's wise to talk all these issues through before you consider moving in together, to develop guidelines that will work for everyone in the family.

Power struggles and control issues can and often do arise in any group of people that live together, whether an extended biological family, a commune, or roommates sharing a flat. These dynamics seem to plague poly families even more than other living groups. This may be because many poly families start with a primary couple. Usually, the initial couple adds another individual, couple, or two individuals to the family unit. Even if the group moves into a neutral space, the couple tends to view themselves as a single unit. Often the couple becomes a voting bloc that can always outnumber the other person(s), or create subtle pressure on the other members. Even the most well-meaning and emotionally healthy couples usually have such a strong bond and so much history together that the other members of the family often feel excluded or overwhelmed. Some poly families have successfully mitigated this problem by having family counseling or mediation to help all partners feel understood, and to resolve outstanding conflicts.

How Can Poly Families Improve Their Chances of Long-Term Sustainability?

Can anything be done to make this poly model more sustainable? Some people blame poly people for being too self-centered or not highly evolved enough to live together successfully. Others suggest that we need training to develop more co-operative living skills, and to learn to be more flexible to accommodate all partners' needs. Some have taken a different approach by suggesting that this model isn't appropriate for most people and needs to be modified to make it work for the masses. They point out that most people who are attempting polyamory are older and somewhat set in their ways, and they may not want to become flexible enough to live with people who have very different diets, habits, and living styles. And most people have little experience in group living, cooperative decision-making, and conflict resolution.

Living with a group requires strong boundaries, interpersonal skills, the ability to articulate your needs clearly, and willingness to compromise. Not everyone wants to take all that on in order to experience the joys of polyamory. In addition, many people have struggled to establish themselves in a profession, save a little money, create a home, and achieve a comfortable standard of living. They may not want to risk everything by merging their finances and living space with other people in a poly family.

One alternative that works for some people involves people living together part-time with some private living space. Variations include two houses on one lot, a duplex, co-housing, or one partner living with each partner half-time in separate households. I call this the "shared custody" model because it is similar to children of divorced parents who live part-time with each parent. These variations are trying for the best of both worlds: They offer the stability and commitment of living together and being a family, and the privacy and autonomy of having your own space. This model allows for a group of people who may not have total compatibility around housework, kids, finances, and living styles to maintain a close, loving, romantic, and family relationship and to sustain it over time.

For example:

Joan and Larry had lived together for eight years when Joan fell in love with Rob. Joan and Larry have good jobs and a beautiful house. They enjoy working on the house, cooking gourmet meals, and collecting fine wines. Rob is a struggling singer-songwriter who lives in a cluttered studio apartment. He rarely cooks or cleans, and lives on frozen burritos, coffee, and cigarettes. He is a recovering alcoholic and does not want any alcohol in his home. Joan wanted Rob to move into their home to create a poly family. Larry knew it wouldn't work because of their incompatible living styles. They worked out an arrangement where Joan spends two weeknights and every Sunday with Rob at his apartment. Most other nights of the week, Rob has dinner with them at their home and then goes home or has music performance gigs, and Joan spends those nights with Larry.

Bill and Esther had been married for six years when Bill met Rachel and developed a committed relationship with her. With Esther's consent, Bill began dividing his time equally between their home and Rachel's home. Rachel had never had children, and at age forty, wanted to have a child with Bill. Esther had raised twins from her previous marriage, and both kids had recently left home to go to college. She was looking forward to some peace and quiet, and did not want to start over with a new baby in the house. They decided to move into a co-housing community where Bill and Esther could have their own house on the same property with Bill and Rachel's house. This way they could all have dinner together every night and spend most of their time together, but have two separate households. Bill continued to spend half of each week living with each partner, and he and Rachel are now expecting a baby.

Elena is a bisexual woman who was living with her lover, Rose, when she got involved with Thomas. After a year, Thomas asked Elena and Rose to move into his large flat. Rose liked Thomas and enjoyed socializing with him, but she is a lesbian and did not want to live with a man. She and Elena were able to find an affordable apartment to rent in the same neighborhood as Thomas. Elena moved some of her clothes, books, and furniture into Thomas' flat, and now spends two days with him, then two days with Rose, etc. She pays rent at both places. She almost moved back in with Rose full-time because Thomas didn't cook or clean house, but he agreed to be more responsible about household chores and she agreed to stay.

Carmen describes herself as "a lesbian with two wives." The three women own a duplex and are on a weekly rotational schedule. Carmen spends three nights each week upstairs with Tanya, and three nights downstairs with Katy. The seventh day of the week is "Carmen's time," and she can negotiate to spend time with either woman if they are available, or to have time to herself. Tanya and Katy each have had outside sexual and romantic relationships, and they see their other girlfriends when Carmen is with the other partner.

Linda has two male spouses, Cliff and Bruce. She co-owns a house with each partner, and lives with each one half-time, changing houses each night. Cliff and Bruce are close friends, but they do not want to live together, as they each prefer to have their own private living space. They are free to pursue relationships with other women if they choose to. Because both men make much higher salaries than Linda and all three have different priorities around money, they have chosen to keep their finances separate. Linda pays one-third of the mortgage, utilities, and other household costs at each house, because she only lives at each house half-time.

Shelley and Ricardo are a married couple from Boston who met Mike and Chandra, a couple from New York, at a Loving More conference six years ago. They got involved and started flying back and forth to spend weekends together. Last year, when Mike and Chandra's daughter left home to go to college, they decided to move to Boston to form a poly family with Shelley and Ricardo. Both couples acknowledged that they were not ready to give up their privacy and having control over their living space, nor were they willing to share their finances. Shelley and Ricardo had a small house on a large lot, so they sold half the lot to Mike and Chandra and they built a small house for themselves. The two couples spend most of their time together, have breakfast and dinner together almost every day. They spend some nights all together sleeping in one room. Other nights they make "dates" with individual partners so that each relationship has time to grow and have privacy. Each couple or any individual can withdraw to their own house if they want time alone or to pursue their own projects. They have discussed the possibility of moving to a bigger house in the future where they would all live together, but they like the benefits of having control over their own space and aren't sure whether that would be better than what they have now.

The "shared custody" model has become more common over the past few years, with more poly relationships in which one or more members live part-time in two households. As you can see from the above examples, this arrangement frequently involves an open "V" triad, where one partner has two primary relationships. Because many people find it logistically challenging and emotionally disorienting to live in two places at once, most people in this model live more in one place than the other. They maintain one primary residence with one spouse, where they receive mail and keep most of their possessions, but they spend a substantial amount of time at the other home as well, usually paying rent and doing chores in both places. A few hardy souls are equally committed to two partners and live equally in two places, dividing their clothes, possessions, time, and financial commitments equally between the two households.

The other most common configuration is two couples that live together most of the time but maintain separate residences, either on the same property or in close proximity.

Taking the Leap Into Living Together?

Anyone forming a poly family would be wise to give careful thought to which model may be most appropriate and satisfying. Be honest with yourself about your needs, about how much privacy and control you are willing to give up, and what you hope to receive from living together as a family. The most important question to ask is, "What could we have by living together that we don't have now, and would we lose anything we now have by moving in together?" If you decide that living together as a group is right for you, it is important to pick partners who are highly compatible and who have group living skills. Make explicit agreements about finances, chore, kids, and privacy before you move in together. If you feel this model may not work for you, consider the "shared custody model" as a possible alternative.

Now that you have learned about the potential joys and pitfalls of living together as a poly family, the next chapter will explore some of the ways in which you can help ensure the legal standing of your poly relationships.

12

Legal Paperwork For Polyamorous Relationships

by Jay Wiseman, JD

Traditional and recognized relationships in a given society have what lawyers sometimes call "standing" — which means that the people in those relationships automatically have certain rights just by the fact that they are in those relationships.

Let's talk a moment about what a "right" is from a lawyer's point of view. In brief, a "right" is a legally enforceable entitlement to do (or refrain from doing) a certain thing. For example, many people in the United States have a right to vote. What that means is that if someone with a right to vote tries to vote, and another person illegally interferes with their doing so, then the wronged person has "standing" (a right) to take their case to court and ask for the court to decree a legally enforceable remedy. "Legally enforceable" means, among other things, that the court-ordered remedy will be enacted by physical force if necessary. The agents of the court will use whatever force is reasonably necessary to carry out the remedy. In the above example, the court's deputies would, if necessary, physically use force to clear the way for the blocked person to have reasonable access to the polls.

In many if not most current societies, traditional relationships, especially very close relationships such as husband/ wife and parent/child, automatically come with certain legally enforceable rights. These rights include the rights to certain property, the right to participate in parenting, the right of visitation if the other person is hospitalized or otherwise institutionalized, and so forth.

Unfortunately, people in non-traditional relationships — including most people in polyamorous relationships — usually do not have such automatically created rights. If a difficulty, such as the death or hospitalization of one partner, takes place, the other partners may find themselves completely shut out by the so-called "real" family; unfortunately the "real" family is often within their rights to enforce their wishes to exclude the nontraditional partners —by force if need be. This can be true even if the partner has been entirely estranged from their "real" family for decades and has been living with their "chosen family" for those decades. "Chosen family members" by and large have no rights at all. This situation, I think we'll all agree, is not good.

Fortunately, it is possible, and generally not all that difficult, to use certain documents to create legal rights for chosen family members that can equal or even exceed those rights that "real" family members have.

Let's look at the Big Issues — illness, death, kids, and property — and how specific documents can be used to create legally enforceable rights for chosen family members.

Illness

The major document that must be created here is called an Advance Healthcare Directive. (Laypeople sometimes call these "living wills," but Advance Healthcare Directive is a more accurate term.) This is basically a document that you create that specifies who you want to make decisions regarding your health care if you become mentally unable to make those decisions for yourself.

Let me make a major point here: Everybody needs one of these documents, even those who are in traditional marriages or legally recognized domestic partnerships. Even if you are married or in a legally recognized domestic partnership and you lose consciousness, then your spouse will not automatically become the decision-maker regarding what should be done — your traditional family members would also have standing to make their thoughts made known to your physicians. If your spouse and your family members disagree as to what should be done regarding your medical care, and you have no advance directive, then your physicians would have to take the matter to court and get a court order regarding how to proceed. The results can be extremely traumatic for those involved. A horrific example of just how bad it can get was provided by the Terri Schiavo case in Florida some years ago, which was dragged through the courts for years.

A basic advance directive names a particular person as the decision-maker regarding healthcare decisions in your stead. It also typically specifies at least one, or possibly two, persons who become the decision-maker if the first person cannot or will not make those decisions. Let me make a major recommendation here: Please do not state that two (or more) people should make these decisions "jointly," because if they disagree, then the matter is once again headed for a court hearing. Legally speaking, it's the better practice to explicitly spell out who is the first person, who is the second person, and who is the third person to be your decision-maker — even if it causes some hurt feelings to do so.

Your Advance Healthcare Directive can cover other matters as well. You may wish to include such items as:

- specific medical treatments that you do and don't want

- instructions that a copy of this directive is to be as enforceable as the original (make sure there is a copy in your doctor's chart)

- who you want to be able to visit you in the hospital (and, if you feel the need, who you don't want to be able to visit you),

- the nomination of a conservator if you are going to need someone to manage your business and financial concerns for a prolonged period of time

- what you want done with your body if you die

- and what arrangements to make regarding your memorial service.

Please note that it's generally better to have matters regarding what to do with your body and your memorial service set forth in your advance directive rather than in your will, because wills often have to go though probate court to be enforced, and that can take weeks or even months. (You can, of course, also mention them in your will if you like.)

Many hospitals and doctors offices have blank advance directive forms that they will give you for the asking. Other documents can be found online. Be advised that their requirements to be legally valid do vary a bit from state to state, so be sure that you create an advance directive that is valid in your particular state. If you move to another state, you should create a new directive.

If you're not in a traditionally recognized relationship, then no matter how many years you have lived together, the hospital staff may refuse to let you visit the person unless you can produce this document.

Also, should you become unconscious or otherwise able to manage your financial affairs, you can create a document that specifies a "durable power of attorney" that allows another person to conduct your financial affairs in your stead. This person could buy and sell property for you, access your bank accounts, and otherwise have access to your financial dealings. Such a document obviously needs to be carefully drafted; if your financial dealings are extensive, you definitely need the advice of an attorney. One type of power of attorney takes effect immediately. Another type is a "springing" durable power of attorney that becomes effective only if, and for as long as, a doctor determines that you are unable to manage your affairs. (You can state your preference in the durable power of attorney as to which doctor you want to make this assessment.)

Death

Many aging boomers are poly, and those boomers are getting old enough to start dying of age-related diseases. Such deaths are starting to happen in significant numbers, and those numbers are only going to increase.

Probably the most stark example of what happens to people in nontraditional families involve the death of one of those family members. Here is where the lack of legal standing can hit especially hard. Basically, if one of your poly family members dies without a will — dies "intestate" — then their legal spouses and/or traditional family members inherit the property they leave behind. The poly family members have absolutely no standing whatsoever to inherit their deceased family member's property — not their personal effects, not their cars, not their real estate — no matter how long they lived together... and no court is likely to grant them standing.

It gets worse. If the deceased person had minor children that the other poly family members were co-parenting, the "real" family is very likely to be able to come in and take the children away until those kids turn eighteen, with the poly family members having zero right of visitation or contact.

Given this very harsh reality, it's truly imperative that people in nontraditional relationships create wills. Wills are especially important if there are particularly expensive items of property to be considered (such as real estate), if there are personal items of particular sentimental value, and, of course, if there minor children are involved.

There are several types of wills. The best type, by far, is a traditional will. This is a will that is typed out, signed and dated by the person creating it (the testator), and signed by at least two "disinterested witnesses" — meaning that the witnesses neither inherit from the will or are involved in either creating it or carrying it out.

There are also handwritten wills — called "holographic" wills — in which all, or at least the most important parts (the "material terms" in legal-speak), are in the testator's handwriting, and the will is signed by the testator. These sorts of wills are only recognized in about half of the states, and even there they are looked at with skepticism because of the obvious potential for fraud. There are other sorts of wills, such as "oral wills" (aka "nuncupative" wills), but these are basically legal curiosities that are only recognized in a very few states and are sharply limited by statute as to what property can be conveyed by them in the few states that do recognize them. Obviously, creating a traditional will is by far the best way to go.

Also, by far the best practice is that a given will cover the estate of only a single person. "Joint wills" (for example, those that cover a husband and wife) are far more subject to ambiguity and challenge. Each person needs their own will.

In a traditional will, you can do a number of things, including but not limited to:

- specify who gets your real property (land and anything permanently attached to that land, such as a house),

- specify who gets your personal property (all property that is not real property),

- nominate a guardian for your children,

- forgive any debts that are owed to you,

- state your wishes regarding what is to be done with your body and what sort of memorial service you want (although these items are, as mentioned above, better handled in your advance directive),

- specify who gets all of your remaining estate.

As mentioned above, your will should be signed by at least two disinterested witnesses. It can be a bit of "cheap insurance" to have a third or even a fourth person sign the will, just in case one of the two original signers doesn't qualify. The signature of the additional witnesses can preserve the will's enforceability. You can also have what's called a "self-proving affidavit" attached to the will. This is a notarized statement that the witnesses were present and saw the testator sign the will. (The notary public will have to actually see the signing of the testator and the witnesses to create this affidavit.) Creating a self-proving affidavit will spare the witnesses from having to appear in probate court to affirm that they saw the testator sign the will.

If there are "big ticket" items involved in the will, such as who gets real estate or who gets nominated as a guardian for the kids, then it's critical that the will be prepared, or at least reviewed, by a poly-friendly attorney licensed in your state to help ensure the will's validity and enforceability. Don't stint on hiring a lawyer and paying for his or her time when something this important is involved.

Several other documents can be created to facilitate the transfer of property upon someone's death. An attorney can talk with you about setting up a trust, creating pay-on-death document with your bank, and other measures relating to your estate and probate court. However, the creation of a valid, enforceable will is by far the single most important step you can take.

Kids

The creation of valid legal paperwork regarding minor children is important. This is especially so if the relationship is in danger of ending, or has already ended, due to death, separation, or other circumstances. Who will handle parenting of the children? Who will pay for their support? Who is entitled to visit them? What rights, if any, do the grandparents have? As mentioned above, one of the most important things that you can do in your will is to nominate a guardian for your kids. This is especially important if you don't want your blood relatives to take over your children's parenting. Fortunately, "parenting agreements" can be created, and are legally enforceable if properly drafted. Other relevant documents can also be created. See the references provided at the end of this article for more specific information.

Property

Whose stuff is it? What belongs to whom? During the course of a relationship, this often isn't all that big a deal; the property is either shared jointly by all, or "everybody knows" what belongs to whom. However, should the relationship end by death or separation, or should a "big ticket" item either come into or leave the relationship (what happens if one of you wins the lottery?), then things can get both angry and muddy very quickly. Some people who are otherwise fairly sane and easygoing can get outright screamingly crazy over money/property issues, and such craziness often doesn't make itself known until one of these issues surfaces.

For example, you've paid for the last four repairs to the car "owned" by one of your poly spouses, and have now put far more into the car than they have. Nothing was ever said about reimbursing you. They then decide to sell the car (their name is the only name on the vehicle's title) and do so for a tidy profit. Are you entitled to any of that money? In the absence of paperwork to the contrary, you may not be. Should you decide to take the matter to court, the judge could quite rationally rule that, in the absence of any agreement otherwise, your paying for the repairs was simply a gift from you to them and therefore not reimbursable.

There are two basic types of property: separate property and community property.

- *Separate property* is property owned by a single person. For example, the computer that I'm writing this article on is my separate property. I can keep it, or sell it, or throw it away, or give it to somebody, and — unless I break a law or something like that — nobody but me has any legally enforceable say in what I do with it.

- *Community property* is property equally owned by two people who are either legally married or in a legally recognized domestic partnership. This means that both people have equal say in what happens to the property — regardless of who earned the money needed to buy it. The general rule is that all income that either party earns during the relationship is community property. (Money or property that comes to one of the partners by means of gift or inheritance is generally the big exception to this community property rule. Money or property acquired by a spouse by gift or inheritance usually remains the separate property of that spouse unless he or she "commingles" it with the community property.) Technically, not a penny of community property money can be spent without the consent of both spouses, nor can community property be sold without the consent of both spouses. While this is generally not enforced regarding small amounts of money or inexpensive items of property, it can be — and sometimes is — enforceable in court regarding large amounts of money or big-ticket items of property. The dissenting spouse often has the legal right to seek, and get, court-ordered reimbursement to the community of the marriage from the other spouse. Also, should one of the spouses die, then the community property automatically becomes owned by the surviving spouse.

- ***Joint property,*** or ***jointly owned property,*** is a third type of property, a form often useful to poly folk. This is property that, by agreement (preferably written agreement), is jointly owned by two, or more, people. In essence, such an agreement turns what would otherwise be separate property into something very similar to community property. It's often wise to include wording to the effect of "this property may not be sold or otherwise transferred without the consent of all owners" in the document. A provision to "buy out" one owner's interest should they decide they no longer want to be part owner of the property can also be included. Also, if the property is jointly owned "with right of survivorship," then the surviving owners automatically become the owners of the property should one of the owners die. (Otherwise, the deceased person's interest may transfer to their heirs.) Obviously, any joint property agreement regarding a big-ticket item should be reviewed by an attorney.

One caution regarding jointly owned property: If one of the owners has significant debts, then the creditors may be able to take over that party's interest in the property. Again, consult an attorney if this is a significant issue.

Poly folk have some other options regarding property ownership. One option is to consider forming a corporation, with the corporation being the actual owner of the property and the poly family members being stockholders in the corporation. Forming such a corporation is not necessarily difficult, but, again, you want to involve a lawyer to make sure that everything is set up properly — especially if big-ticket items are involved.

Moving Forward

The most important thing you can do about all these documents is to actually create them. Many people "have been meaning to get around to" creating such documents, but it keeps getting put off — and then, when a tragedy strikes, it's usually too late. I've designated my birthday, June 16th, as "check your preparations" day. On that day I recommend that people review their emergency training (is their CPR card current?), their emergency equipment (where are those fire extinguishers and first aid kits?), and their emergency paperwork (where are the advance healthcare directive and the wills?).

It's important to store your truly urgent emergency paperwork — especially your advance healthcare directive and your will — in a place where it can be reached quite readily. In particular, lawyers recommend that you do not store them in a safe deposit box. Safe deposit boxes can be difficult for others to get into if you're in the hospital, and if you die then the box may be sealed until ordered open by the court. Instead, take a large envelope, perhaps red in color or otherwise made easy to find, and place it somewhere in your house. Copies of your advance healthcare directive can also be left with your doctor's chart and in other places. Some companies offer online "safes" where you can store backups of these papers, and where you can designate who is allowed to access them.

Poly organizations can hold an annual "get your paperwork in order" day that can be devoted to this topic. Blank documents, such as advance healthcare directives, can be distributed at such events. If possible, have one or more attorneys who are knowledgeable in this area attend to answer questions. "Legal paperwork" programs can also be presented at large poly gatherings.

Further information can be found online. Just type "estate planning" into a search engine and you'll find numerous resources. One particularly good resource is Nolo Press — www.nolo.com — which offers online information and many useful books regarding estate planning, family law, and so forth.

In summary, poly folk and other people in non-traditional relationships generally have no legally enforceable rights, but a few documents — that can generally be created with fairly minimal fuss or expense — can create such rights. Make sure you get around to doing so before it's too late.

PART FIVE
Special Issues and Topics

13
Navigating Polyamorous BDSM Relationships

Many people have noticed that there is a fair amount of overlap between the group of people who have a BDSM orientation and those who have multiple relationships or practice some form of polyamory. BDSM or sadomasochism practitioners enjoy one or more form of "kink" as part of their erotic and intimate life, such as bondage, pain play or impact play, dominance and /or submission, fetishes, role playing, or "master/slave" or "mistress/slave" relationships. While many who enjoy and practice some form of BDSM are strictly monogamous, a significant percentage are in open relationships of some type and have multiple partners. There are a lot of reasons for this overlap in the two affinities or orientations. And while in many ways polyamory fits well with BDSM, it can also create some unique and very challenging problems.

Why Do Kinky People Want Open Relationships?

As mentioned in Chapter 1, poly people in general want either More or Different. If they are looking for More, they may want more romance, attention, sex, or time than they can have with their current partner. If instead they want Different, one or more crucial ingredients are missing from their current relationship that really would make them happier, so they are seeking those ingredients from someone else.

Kinky people who are poly tend to be looking for Different rather than More. Usually they are looking for something kinky that their partner doesn't want to do, either because their partner is not kinky, or their partner likes a different kind of BDSM activity than they do. Some people simply have a strong need for novelty and variety in sexual and BDSM partners.

As most kinky people have discovered, it is difficult to find the partner that is perfectly matched with your core kinks, as well as compatible for a long-term relationship and living together. Often your best kink partner is not your best marriage or life partner; as a result, people tend to marry or live with people who are well-suited to be their domestic partners, but look outside the primary relationship for BDSM activity with others who are more closely matched with their BDSM needs.

Why Do Kinky People Tend to Be More Successful In Polyamorous Relationships?

It is clear, in my experience, that people with a BDSM orientation tend to be more successful at establishing and sustaining polyamorous relationships than vanilla or non-kinky people. While of course many vanilla people are quite talented and successful at poly relationships, a higher percentage of BDSM poly relationships succeed over time than vanilla BDSM relationships.

At first this gap may seem puzzling. However, it makes perfect sense that kinky people in general are better at polyamory than vanilla people in general for two important reasons:

-   In many BDSM relationships, each person's role and rights are clearly defined and delineated in some detail. As any veteran of poly relationships can attest, conflicts over roles, status, rights, and responsibilities are often the snags that cause many poly relationships to crash and burn. In BDSM relationships, on the other hand, often each person has a specific set of roles, has a clearly defined status, and knows what is expected of them and what they have a right to expect of each other person. For instance, if you are in a D/S relationship, your role as a submissive is clearly spelled out, and you and your dominant have negotiated exactly what you are to provide for the dom and exactly what she or he is expected to provide for you. Your status in relation to your partner(s) and your partner's other partners is also clearly agreed upon, so there is less room for assumptions and misunderstandings about your status and the hierarchy of relationships. In many vanilla poly relationships, unstated and unmet expectations create a lot of pain.

- The skill set needed for successful BDSM relationships is also essential for successful polyamorous relationships. In Parts Two and Three of this book, we discussed many of the components of the skill set required for successful polyamory. Many of these skills are also necessary for successful BDSM relationships. Most important are:
  a) Knowing what you want.
  b) Being able and willing to articulate your needs clearly. People in BDSM relationships have wisely abandoned the romantic myth that relationships will go perfectly without discussion and negotiation. They have institutionalized negotiations as part of their courtship and relationship rituals.
  c) Willingness to negotiate, including being able to set boundaries and knowing how to compromise.
  d) Not making assumptions about your partner's desires, needs, expectations, and abilities.
  e) Not expecting a partner to read your mind and magically know what you want.

How can you increase the odds of successful and happy kinky/poly relationships?

- ***Pick appropriate partners.*** Many people make the mistake of picking partners who are poly but are not kinky. Even if you're compatible on poly issues, if your partner does not share your BDSM orientation, a relationship is unlikely to be sustainable over time. Some mixed couples where one is kinky and the other is vanilla build poly relationships in which the kinky partner has permission to do BDSM activities with outside partners. Sometimes, such couples agree that only non-sexual kink activities with outside partners are acceptable, and that sex will be exclusive to the primary relationship. (Such couples must negotiate their own definitions of what constitutes "sex.")

Others are comfortable with their partners having sex activities with other partners.

It is also a mistake to pick partners who are kinky but are not poly. Sometimes this can work if a non-poly submissive is comfortable allowing their dominant to be poly, seeing their own commitment to be monogamous as part of being submissive. Typically, in this situation, the dominant partner has other sexual partners and/or submissives, but the sub agrees to be monogamous. However, many submissives are not willing to agree to this arrangement and feel very threatened by their partner dominating anyone else or having a sexual relationship with anyone outside the primary relationship. This can be a deal-breaker if the dominant partner feels they have the right to have outside partners, and the submissive partner insists on monogamy.

Most people do not get it right the first time, and need to go through a few relationships, and some trial and error, to learn what does and doesn't work for them.

- ***Know which model of polyamory you are in,*** and pick appropriate partners who match that model. As was discussed extensively in Chapter Two, it is imperative that you figure out which model of polyamory works best for you and pick partners that are looking for the same model. This is even more true for BDSM relationships, because of the explicit roles and hierarchy in kinky relationships. For instance, if you decide on the primary/secondary model, you would be wise to pick a primary partner who wants a long-term, committed relationship and wants only secondary partners outside your relationship. You would also be smart to choose outside partners who are also in primary relationships or who are looking for a casual or secondary relationship rather than seeking a primary relationship with you.

Conversely, if you are looking for a committed primary relationship, it would be disastrous to pick someone who is already married and not looking for an additional spouse.

Unfortunately many people pick partners who want a different model, and make each other miserable by trying to force their partners to accept a model that doesn't work for them.

- ***Expect and learn to handle jealousy,*** both yours and your partner's. The vast majority of people experience jealousy when their partners get involved in a romantic, sexual and/or BDSM relationship with someone else. As discussed in Part Four of this book, sharing our partner's time, attention, loyalty, and sexual intimacy with another person represents a potential threat to the survival and stability of our precious love relationship. It is natural to respond with concern and anxiety. Try to be caring and compassionate with yourself and your partner(s) through this process, expressing feelings and fears, listening carefully to your partner's feelings and needs, and trying to support each other. For a more complete guide to handling jealousy, you can review Part Four and/or read some of the books on jealousy described in the "More Resources" section at the end of this book.

Some Specific Tips for Working With Jealousy in BDSM/Poly Relationships

Try to identify exactly what triggers your jealousy. Some people discover that they are much more jealous of a partner engaging in BDSM activities with another partner than having sex with another partner. This is because for some people, specific types of BDSM activities are even more personal and intimate than sex.

For example:

Mae, a dominant woman, was extremely hurt and jealous that her submissive Ed wanted to participate in "humiliation" scenes with another woman. While these scenes did not involve any sexual contact, they included Ed being extremely submissive; Mae felt threatened by the level of intimacy and vulnerability Ed was willing to experience with another woman. She wanted these experiences to be "special" and exclusively in their relationship. She had no problem with Ed performing sexual acts with another person, as she did not feel this was as unique and personal as the BDSM experiences which she wanted him to reserve only for her.

Billie and Violet, a lesbian couple who enjoyed flogging and other impact play, discovered that they each became extremely jealous when their partner wore their leather and fetish clothing or used their floggers or toys on another woman. Both women felt that their BDSM clothes and toys were special to that relationship and should not be used outside the relationship.

Other people find that they area very comfortable with their partners doing many types of BDSM activities with outside partners but want to reserve sex (or certain types of sexual activities) to the primary relationship. Some people find it easy to separate sex and BDSM, and compartmentalize some BDSM activities in outside relationships that do not include sex.

However, for many people, sex and BDSM are difficult to separate and keep neatly in separate relationships. Jealousy and conflict may ensue if a couple agrees to sexual monogamy but their outside BDSM activities tend to lead to sex, or conversely if outside sexual relationships inevitably lead them into BDSM activities.

Be clear on your role in each relationship, what role you want from each partner, and negotiate to change those roles if your needs or desires change. This is especially important in BDSM relationships, because something that starts out as a casual "play partner" relationship can rapidly become a dom-sub relationship or even a master- or mistress-slave relationship. As a result, any or all partners can be hurt or disappointed if their escalating expectations are not met.

When one or more partners are switches and want to change or alternate roles in one or more relationships, more discussion and negotiation is always better than less, to clarify and define needs, expectations, and boundaries.

Having too many doms in a given poly relationship grouping can be a thorny problem, as it is difficult to know who has authority to tell whom to do what. Establishing a clear hierarchy of all existing relationships at the beginning of each relationship is crucial, as is clarifying matters immediately if anyone's status changes.

Clearly defining what each partner means by the terms they use is also imperative. Terms like top, dom, and master or mistress, bottom, submissive, and slave can mean very different things to each person. While there are no universally agreed-upon definitions, it doesn't matter how you define them as long as everyone in the relationship grouping is working with the same definitions.

When problems develop in a BDSM/poly relationship, the bottom line is usually this: will being poly trump the BDSM role, or will BDSM trump being poly? Essentially it boils down to this: are you more kinky or more poly? Is BDSM your primary sexual orientation, and it that central to your relationship "world view," or is polyamory your primary orientation and will that be the arbiter of how you want to do relationships? Some people find that their poly and BDSM orientations are roughly equal, and they must decide on a case by case basis, depending on the relationship and the specifics of that situation.

Some examples of BDSM/poly dilemmas, and some potential solutions:

Jen is a dom in a primary relationship with Bonnie, who is a sub. Bonnie also subs to her secondary partner, Donna. When Bonnie is at a play party with Jen, Donna feels hurt because she can't interact with her, as Bonnie is sitting at Jen's feet and is subbing to her. Bonnie feels torn because Donna is also her dom, and she wants to show deference to her, but that intrudes on the boundaries of her D/S relationship with Jen.

How can they solve this problem? Jen could give Bonnie permission to interact with Donna and sub to her at play parties for a specific time limit, such as for fifteen or thirty minutes at the beginning or end of the party or while Jen is playing with someone else. Or Jen could devise scenes in which Donna would be the "middle," domming Bonnie under Jen's direction. Another option would be for Bonnie to accompany Donna to certain play parties which Jen would not attend. Parties where Bonnie was with Jen would either be off-limits to Donna (she would agree to miss those parties) or she could agree not to approach Bonnie or expect interaction with her at these specific events.

Another problem is that when Bonnie is at Donna's home with her and is in sub space, Jen often calls by phone and demands her attention. Jen feels since she is the primary dom, she has the right to trump Bonnie's time with Donna and interrupt at any time. Because they are poly, Bonnie feels she has the right to uninterrupted sub space with Donna. One option would be for Bonnie to agree to call Jen at least once while at Donna's house, but to do so only after asking permission from Donna to come out of role, and going into a different room in the house to make the call. Or, Jen can approach Donna "dom to dom" and negotiate an agreement about when phone calls will be made.

Each of these solutions assumes that Jen and Bonnie's relationship is equally poly and kinky. If their orientation is more kinky than poly, a different approach is necessary. Jen might insist that Bonnie end her relationship with Donna because it impedes her ability to be completely submissive to Jen. Or Donna might decide that the polyamorous aspect of her relationship with Bonnie prevents Bonnie from being available enough to be her submissive and comply with her requests. As a result, Donna may end the relationship and seek out a single submissive who can have a full-time D/S relationship.

Charles and Melinda identify as being in a mistress/slave relationship. Charles has been collared to Melinda for ten years, and they have been living together for eight years. They are polyamorous and Melinda is a switch. Melinda has a mistress, Athena, to whom she subs. However, when Melinda subs to Athena, Charles feels abandoned and unsafe, and feels his mistress is not available to him to provide a safe container for his submission. Melinda feels he is being manipulative and immature, but in fact he has a legitimate dilemma shared by many subs whose doms are switches. It is very challenging for a sub, especially a slave, to feel safe if their dom temporarily shifts from being in control and subs to someone else.

One option for resolving this problem is for Charles to accompany Melinda or be present when she subs to Athena, and for Athena to create a safe space for Charles and be responsible for him as his temporary mistress while Melinda is in sub space. Another approach is for Melinda to ask another dom that she trusts to be in charge of Charles temporarily while she is with Athena, *so Charles will feel taken care of and will have the attention and direction he craves. These solutions assume that each relationship is more fundamentally kinky and less poly, so the primary goal is to satisfy the sub's need for submission and the dom's need for control. If the core orientation of each of these individuals were more poly than kinky, then Melinda may insist that Charles do some personal growth work to become more self-sufficient, such as going to counseling or to poly support groups, so that he can manage his feelings and take care of himself during times when she is not available to direct him. Or Charles could develop his own outside relationship with another mistress who he could sub to when Melinda is with Athena.*

Peter and Tom have lived together for 15 years. Their relationship started out kinky only in the bedroom, and was egalitarian and vanilla outside of the sexual relationship. Peter is a sadist and expert in bondage and discipline, and Tom loves stringent bondage and frequent floggings. Peter also enjoys electricity play with the violet wand, but Tom is totally freaked out by it, so Peter practices this particular activity with many other men. Tom likes age play but Peter is uncomfortable with it because he was molested by a priest in childhood, so Tom does occasional age play with two other older men. Over the years their primary relationship has developed into a 24/7 D/S relationship, and now they both have developed some intense jealousy and feelings of betrayal whenever the other plays with someone else. Peter is pressuring Tom to drop the two other "daddies" and be monogamous with him.

This is a frequent dilemma in D/S poly relationships: many doms believe that it is their right to have outside partners but that their submissive partner should be monogamous. Some subs are very happy with this arrangement and see being monogamous with a non-monogamous partner as part of their submission. However, submissives whose core orientation is polyamorous may not be willing to be monogamous, creating an intense conflict over relationship roles and boundaries.

Some pairings solve this problem by making very specific rules about what kind of play is permitted outside of the primary relationship. Some decide that only BDSM activity is allowed outside of the relationship, and that no overtly sexual activity is allowed. Some limit the activities only to BDSM activities that are not practiced within the relationship. For example, Tom is only allowed to do age play with other men, while other types of BDSM and other sexual activities are exclusively practiced between Peter and Tom. And Peter is only allowed to use the wand on other men, and all other sexual or BDSM activities are reserved for Tom.

If Peter and Tom's orientation were more kinky than poly, Tom might agree to drop the two other lovers and be monogamous with Peter. Peter may try to meet Tom's desire for age play by taking him to play parties and ordering him to do age play with other men at the parties, under his direction and control.

Fern is in a mistress/slave relationship with her wife Andrea, and they have been together 13 years. Andrea enjoys being caned and flogged; she loves impact play and needs a high level of pain. Fern has always enjoyed providing this for her. However, she recently developed carpal tunnel syndrome in her wrists due to working at a computer all day at her job, and her doctor advised her to stop doing flogging and caning for six months to allow healing.

Fern gave Andrea permission to be flogged by their friend Dolores, another mistress with a firm hand. However, Andrea and Dolores have now developed a loving and sexual relationship and Fern feels jealous and betrayed. (As in any poly relationship, what starts off casual and friendly can rapidly escalate to falling in love.)

These three women have a few choices: Andrea may have to end the relationship with Dolores because it is threatening the primary relationship between Andrea and Fern, and instead get caning and flogging either at play parties from casual partners or with partners that are picked and/or supervised by Fern. Or Andrea and Dolores may agree to have only a BDSM relationship involving impact play but no sex, and see if they can step back from the romantic relationship. Or Fern may explore her jealousy through poly workshops, counseling or help from other poly people or support networks, and learn to feel secure enough to allow Andrea to have a strong sexual and romantic bond with Dolores.

As you can see, people with a BDSM orientation face some unique challenges in navigating open relationships. However, as we have discussed, kinky people tend to be very successful at developing and sustaining polyamorous relationships. This is because clear communication, negotiating boundaries, and explicitly identifying rights and expectations are a core component to BDSM relationships. For people to succeed in kinky relationships, they must develop the same skill set necessary for healthy open relationships.

Sex Addiction and Polyamory, and How to Tell the Difference

Are Polyamorous People Really Just a Bunch of Sex Addicts?

Polyamorous people have become accustomed to people confusing us with sex addicts, or accusing us of being sex, love, and relationship addicts. Many people erroneously believe that if someone has more than one sexual or romantic partner concurrently, they must be a sex addict. If we try to explain that polyamory is not just about sex, it is about loving more, then they accuse us of being love and relationship addicts.

On the other hand, many polyamorous people believe that the very concept of sex addiction is just a sex-negative backlash being promoted by monogamists who seek to pathologize polyamory. Many polyamorous people do not believe that sex addiction really exists, but rather that it is a convenient fiction to attack those of us who do not conform to traditional models of sexual behavior. In my professional experience as a counselor and my personal experience as a polyamorous woman for nearly forty years, I have seen many happy healthy polyamorists and I have seen many *bona fide* sex and relationship addicts.

It is important to understand both sex addiction and love and relationship addiction, for at least two reasons. First of all, being knowledgeable allows us to articulately counter accusations that all poly people are addicts. Second, if we know and recognize the signs and symptoms of sex and relationship addiction, we can avoid getting involved with addicted people, and can identify any potentially compulsive or unhealthy behaviors in ourselves.

Some people who claim to be polyamorous really *are* sex or relationship addicts, using polyamory as a philosophical excuse to act out compulsive and destructive relationship patterns. Just as some people choose monogamy for unhealthy reasons or to hide their dysfunctional relationship behaviors, people may choose polyamory as a cover-up for their addictive behavior. People who have an addictive relationship with sex or love make very poor relationship partners in general, and they are not good candidates for successful poly relationships. They are too self-centered and too caught up in their own addictive disease to be capable of real intimacy or of truly loving anyone.

If you recognize the warning signs, you can save yourself and your other partners a lot of grief by avoiding involvement with people suffering from sex or love addiction. If you recognize some of these traits in yourself or in someone you are involved with already, you can minimize the damage to yourself and your relationships by seeking counseling or other types of healing support.

What Are Sex and Love Addiction?

Sex addiction and love and relationship addiction are two sides of the same coin, the same disease manifested in two different ways.

- *Sex addiction* is a compulsive need to engage in very frequent sexual activity with many partners, and a belief that pursuing and procuring sex is the number one priority in life. Sex addicts feel driven to pursue any and all sexual feelings and attractions they experience, without thinking through the pros and cons of the particular situation. Sex is the only thing that creates feelings of comfort and satisfaction in their lives, and they experience sex as a "high," like a drug. They feel powerful in their lives only when having sex, and they feel alive only when pursuing or having sex. Their desire for more sex with more partners often clouds their judgment and they will do almost anything to manipulate people into sex. They often violate their own values and break existing agreements with partners in order to get more sex, usually lying in order to cover up their betrayals. They use sex very much as other addicts use drugs or alcohol: to experience an intense high they can't get any other way, to distract themselves from boredom and anxiety, and/or to numb loneliness and emotional pain. Like other addictions, sex addiction is a progressive disease that worsens over time. At first a sex addict will bend the rules and break minor agreements with partners, stretching the truth but not overtly lying. The addict may try to exercise some restraint to avoid sexual situations which are sure to have disastrous consequences. But eventually, they take more and more risks, engaging in very dangerous sexual behaviors regardless of the consequences. Finally they lose all self-respect, as well as the respect of their partners, because of their lying and inability to keep any agreements they have made.

- *Love and relationship addiction* manifests in a different way. Instead of being primarily focused on sex, a love and relationship addict is excessively dependent on being in love and being in a relationship. Love addicts organize their lives around their relationships and sacrifice their own needs, their careers, their health, and even their self-respect in order to stay in relationships, no matter how badly they are treated. Their self-esteem and identity are heavily dependent on the relationship, and they believe that they could not survive without it. Their attachment to their relationship partners provides their only sense of being valuable and worthwhile human beings.

Currently, the majority of sex addicts are men, and most love and relationship addicts are women. Why is this? Men and women are socialized in very different ways in our society. Men are taught to prioritize sex and women are trained to value relationships over all else. And recent research indicates that men and women may be "wired" very differently in their sexual desires and sexual response, as well as in their experience of sex and relationships. Sex hormones such as testosterone, estrogen, and progesterone may play a greater role than previously believed.

The jury is still out on the "nature vs. nurture" controversy, but at this point in history, for whatever reason, men are much more likely to use sex addictively, while women are much more likely to become addicted to love and relationships.

What's the Difference Between Polyamory and Sex Addiction?

Healthy poly people prioritize sex and intimate relationships in their lives, and devote a significant amount of time and energy to creating and sustaining sexual and romantic relationships. Some focus more attention on emotional intimacy and relationships, while others are more oriented towards recreational sex and emphasize sex more than long-term relationships. However, despite our focus on sex and/or relationships, we are not addicted to sex or relationships.

I sometimes use humor to explain that I am a "sex maniac, not a sex addict," and I often describe myself as a "relationship enthusiast" rather than a love and relationship addict. I use the terms "sex maniac" and "relationship enthusiast" as I feel they convey that I value sex and relationships and make them a priority in my life. However, sex and love are not the only focus in my life, and I have a fulfilling and well-rounded life outside of relationships. Sex and relationships enhance my quality of life and bring me physical, emotional, and spiritual satisfaction. I find that intense and loving relationships and sex make me a warmer, more compassionate, and more open person in every other area of my life. However, I am a whole person on my own, and could live a happy and meaningful life without sex and relationships.

Being a sex maniac involves being "sex-positive," seeing sex and sexuality as a positive force, and rejecting negative beliefs about sex being shameful or wrong. I am a relationship enthusiast because connecting lovingly with others gives me a deeper understanding of people and encourages me to pursue needed personal growth, to know myself better and become a more loving person. However, I know that even without romantic relationships, life would still be vibrant and delightful, and I would focus on other meaningful experiences and activities that are equally valid. Since I feel secure that I am a lovable and valuable person, I don't need to constantly validate my desirability through sexual or romantic conquests, as sex and love addicts feel compelled to do.

So the difference between polyamorists and sex addicts is approximately equal to the difference between social drinkers and alcoholics. Social drinkers can enjoy a few drinks or a glass of wine to socialize with friends or relax at home after work, and they make responsible choices about when, where, what, and how much to drink. And they can enjoy life without drinking, and will not become anxious and depressed if there is no alcohol available. Poly people enjoy sex and relationships, and we usually exercise good judgment about whom to get involved with and under what conditions, what kind of relationships to have, and how many sexual relationships we can handle at one time.

Some Examples of Sex and Love Addiction

The main differences between polyamory and sex or relationship addiction are the addicts' lack of control over their behavior and their inability to make rational choices about sex and relationships.

For example:

Alan is a heterosexual man who identifies as poly. He has been married and divorced twice, both times to poly women. In his first marriage he made unwelcome sexual advances to every one of his wife's female friends, and eventually she lost all her friends because they got tired of being sexually harassed by him. His first wife left him because he spent half his paycheck every month on prostitutes and phone sex. During his second marriage, he again tried to seduce his wife's friends, even after agreeing to her request that he only have sex with women outside of their immediate social circle. His second wife left after he was fired from his job for taking three-hour lunches to go to strip clubs and massage parlors.

George is a straight man in a poly marriage with his wife; he also has an outside lover he sees a few times a week. Despite having sex every day with his wife and/or his lover, he feels compelled to cruise the Internet seeking additional sex partners. He ignores his work at the office and spends hours a day surfing the Web trying to meet women for sex. He has lost several jobs because his productivity is significantly lowered by the time he spends in the Internet looking for sex. He met two young women through posting an ad for a job for fashion models, and manipulated them into sex by falsely implying that he could get them modeling jobs. Although he suspected that they were underage, he pressured them into sex anyway, and eventually ended up in jail for having sex with minors.

Lisa is a bisexual poly woman in a primary relationship with a man. She likes to go dancing at clubs and pick up both male and female partners, and she often goes to sex parties to meet sex partners. She has such a strong compulsion to have sex that she often makes poor partner choices and goes home with questionable and even dangerous men. She drinks alcohol and often makes decisions while under the influence, and frequently forgets to use birth control and condoms for safer sex. She has accidentally gotten pregnant twice and had two abortions; she has had gonorrhea and chlamydia. She was beaten and robbed by one man she picked up at a party, even though other women at the party were suspicious of him and warned her to avoid him. Despite these consequences, she continues to engage in risky behaviors without thinking through possible ways to create safer conditions to enjoy her sexual freedom.

Dina is a lesbian who is a love and relationship addict. She had a relationship for several years with a woman who was very controlling, was jealous of her friends, and who didn't want her to visit or talk to her family. Although they had agreed to an open relationship, and her partner had other girlfriends from time to time, whenever Dina was interested in dating others, her partner always found a reason to veto them. Dina turned over her paycheck to her partner every month and allowed her to make most decisions in the relationship. She was very unhappy but was afraid to express her needs or concerns. She felt she couldn't leave because she felt her only value as a person was in being in a relationship, and felt terrified of being alone.

John is a bisexual man in a committed primary relationship with a man, and both are poly. John has had a long series of outside relationships with other men, and each one follows the same pattern: He meets someone new and immediately falls madly in love, jumping into an intense romantic relationship for a few months. Then, as the infatuation starts to wear off and he gets to know the person, he loses interest and breaks up with the new lover. Soon he starts looking around for someone else, because he is addicted to the fantasy and romance of New Relationship Energy and has to get another "fix."

Jason is a heterosexual college professor. He and his wife were in a poly relationship and both dated other partners. However, his wife eventually left him because he consistently picked inappropriate partners. He repeatedly had brief, intense affairs with his students, who were thirty years younger than he, because he needed constant validation that women found him desirable. Because Jason was addicted to relationships where he could feel powerful and be worshipped, he consistently picked naïve, vulnerable, teen-aged women who would fall in love with him and become very dependent on him. Of course, as soon as each woman began to assert her own needs, he ended the relationship and moved on to his next victim.

Lorraine is a heterosexual poly woman. She lives alone but has three male lovers and sees each one approximately two nights a week. Despite having sex nearly every day with one of her partners, she is not sexually satisfied and masturbates daily. She pressures her lovers for sex even if they are tired or sick with the flu, and becomes depressed and angry if they say no.

Huey is a sex addict who had a poly relationship with his wife until she divorced him. Both are heterosexual and enjoyed "swing parties," but he became sullen and withdrawn if he didn't "score" sexually at every party. He frequently pressured his wife into having sex with men she did not feel comfortable with, just so he would be allowed to sleep with their wives. He became coercive and threatening if she didn't consent. When his wife was quite ill during a pregnancy, she felt very vulnerable and asked him to refrain from having other partners for a few months until she had the baby. He refused to honor her request and immediately placed his profile on a dating website and began having an affair with another woman for the duration of the pregnancy.

Facilitating Positive Change

I have worked with many sex, love and relationship addicts who have decided to work on their issues and develop healthier beliefs and behaviors. If they are unhappy with the problems their addictions are causing them in their lives, and are willing to seek out help, they can dramatically improve their relationship patterns. Individual counseling or hypnotherapy can help people understand how they developed these beliefs and attitudes in the first place, and how they can meet their sexual and relationship needs in a healthier way. Couples or family counseling can also be helpful in rebuilding trust between partners and undoing whatever damage the addiction has done in current relationships.

Joining a polyamory support group or discussion group or going on-line to talk to other poly people can help people differentiate between addictive and healthy behaviors and provide positive role models of healthy poly relationships. There are twelve-step recovery groups called Sex and Love Addicts Anonymous (SLAA), based on the Alcoholics Anonymous model, and free, confidential meetings of these groups are available in most cities. Many sex and love addicts find these groups extremely helpful in learning new skills and attitudes about sex and relationships. However, some people experience these meetings as sex-negative, or complain that many people in twelve-step groups are hostile to open relationships. People often have to try a few different kinds of groups before finding one that meets their needs.

In addition, a number of excellent books have been written on sex addiction in recent years. These can be an important resource for people trying to understand and change their addictive patterns in relationships.

The issue of sex and love addiction is very controversial within the polyamorous community and discussion on this subject is ongoing.

15

When You Are the Outside Relationship: A Brief Guide to Being a "Secondary Partner"

Most of this book has been focused on couples in primary relationships, since most open relationships start out with a primary couple and expand from there to include outside relationships. But what if you are the outside relationship or the so-called "secondary" partner? How can you navigate this very confusing and sometimes painful experience of being involved with someone who is already committed to another relationship which they explicitly identify as primary? This chapter will give you some guidance on managing the complex array of feelings and dilemmas that are most commonly experienced by secondary partners.

People who are already in a primary relationship and are looking for another relationship are the most likely to be happy in the role of secondary partner. Secondary relationships are also a good fit for people who have another overriding commitment in their lives that is so absorbing and time-consuming that a primary relationship is not practical or desirable.

For example:

Hannah is a single parent with two teenage daughters, Janet is a folk musician and music producer that tours ten months out of the year, Jill is a scientist doing intensive research for a cure for AIDS, and David is a political activist that is in meetings every night until 11 PM. Each of them is in a secondary relationship, each with a lover who is married to someone else. This arrangement works well for them because they can have love and companionship in their lives without diverting much time and attention away from their "mission" of raising kids, making music, or saving the world.

Yvonne and Martin are happily married. Yvonne enjoys having a casual or dating relationship with someone outside her primary relationship. Most of her needs for companionship, intimacy, and sex are met in her marriage, and she devotes the bulk of her free time to that relationship. She got involved in a secondary relationship with Jim, who is also married and in a poly relationship with his wife. They have dates once a week on Thursday nights when Martin works late and doesn't get home until midnight, so it doesn't cut into their time together. Once a month they get together on a Saturday or Sunday because Jim's wife spends those weekends visiting her elderly mother. Both Yvonne and Jim prioritize their spouses and children over the secondary relationship, and both are comfortable with the explicit limits of the relationship.

What Can Go Wrong

Even a seemingly perfect secondary relationship can go awry. Something that started as casual can become an intense love affair and begin to take too much time and emotional commitment away from the primary relationship. Or someone who was completely absorbed with something else suddenly becomes more available for a primary relationship.

Sometimes this happens because the secondary relationship is free of the constraints of everyday life. The relationship with the secondary partner is fun dates and romance, with none of the everyday drudgery of negotiations about chores, bills, work, and kids. This situation can create the illusion that the primary relationship is all work and the secondary relationship is all play. It's hard for a long-term relationship to compete with the "shiny new toy" aspect of a new relationship.

Many people in this situation find themselves comparing the carefree dinner dates and passionate trysts they enjoy with their secondary partner with doing housework, getting the kids to bed, and falling into bed exhausted with their spouse.

If you find yourself in this situation, it is important to remember that you are comparing apples and oranges. The secondary relationship is new and unknown and there is no security or certainty that it will continue, while the long-term partnership is stable and comfortable.

Each relationship has its strengths. The beauty of polyamory is that you can have your cake and eat it too: you can have the excitement and romance of a new relationship without giving up the security and intimacy of a stable life partnership. Both are precious and can be managed concurrently. The pitfall is in confusing the two and mistakenly thinking that the hot new love affair should eclipse the primary relationship.

If you think back to when you first were dating your spouse, you will remember that it was just as exciting and romantic as your secondary relationship is now, if not more so. While the sizzle of passion will inevitably cool somewhat as you get to know the real person and commit to a long-term partnership, a little less lust and romance leads to a lot more stability and true intimacy. Don't take your partner for granted and delude yourself that you will be happier leaving your spouse for the secondary partner, no matter how tempting that may seem when passions are high. This fantasy may be a sign that you need to pay more attention to your primary relationship and nurture the spark of romance by making special dates or spending more quality time together. Or there may be some issues in your primary relationship that are creating some distance or dissatisfaction, and need to be addressed. You may benefit from reading Chapter 10 , "Are You In Poly Hell?," for a more detailed discussion of this phenomenon and the danger signs of demotion, displacement, and intrusion.

When It Isn't Enough

Sometimes a secondary relationship can be very painful if you are really seeking a primary relationship and want more than this relationship can provide. Often it is not so much a choice as a coincidence. You meet someone and are attracted to each other, but you discover that he or she is already in a committed polyamorous relationship. Your potential partner offers you only two options: enter the relationship as a secondary partner or walk away. You do not have the leverage to change the rules and limits that have already been established in the primary relationship. Many people are so drawn to someone that they get romantically involved even though the conditions of the relationship are not ideal for them.

For example:

Justin is a single heterosexual man in a secondary relationship with Trina, who is in a primary relationship with Joaquin. At first Justin thought this was too good to be true: a casual relationship with a woman who loved sex and didn't make any demands on him for attention or commitment. However, after a year of seeing Trina one night a week and having occasional weekends together, he was in love and wanted more. She negotiated with Joaquin to have one additional night with Justin every other week, but he balked at their rules and felt neglected and disrespected. Eventually he left the relationship because he could not get his needs met within the boundaries of the secondary relationship.

Natalie is a 35-year-old single bisexual woman who got involved in a relationship with a married couple, Paul and Ayisha. She met them at a bisexual brunch event, they invited her to their home for dinner and ended up in bed together. She was just exploring her own bisexual feelings after her divorce, and wasn't expecting to get involved with anyone. She recalls, "It was like a freak accident. I met them and was absolutely smitten, I was so confused because I had never been attracted to two people at the same time, and never had a relationship with a woman. I fell totally in love with them, but they wanted something casual, as their relationship was primary. I was crushed as I had no experience with polyamory, and I wanted to be with them all the time." They spent every other weekend together as a threesome, and developed an intense bond during their year-long courtship. Their dates were incredibly satisfying and pleasurable, but Natalie was lonely all week long when they were not together. She pleaded for more time and commitment, and Paul was open to her becoming a primary partner, but Ayisha felt threatened and convinced Paul that they should end the relationship with Natalie. She was devastated, as she was deeply in love with them both.

While it is perfectly reasonable to want more time and attention, and to want equality, this change in the agreement requires the consent of everyone in the relationship. In this case, Ayisha feared that Natalie's real agenda was to displace her and become Paul's primary partner, and insisted they end the relationship.

This situation is unfortunately only too common among poly people, as people often follow their hearts and their libido instead of their heads. It may be tempting to believe that you can live with your partner's limits, even if that means only seeing him once every two weeks on a weeknight. You may think you can tolerate never spending the night with your partner, if that is the rule in her primary relationship. However, the reality may create loneliness and anger, and you may feel mistreated, unloved, and abandoned. You may feel panic when you need contact with your lover and you are not allowed to call him at home when he is with his primary partner. You may experience rage and despair when your partner cancels dates with you because her husband is feeling insecure and wants her to stay at home with him that night, or if a family event comes up which trumps your date.

The crux of the problem for most secondary partners hinges on two problems: the scarcity of time, attention, and contact, which leads to a chronic experience of deprivation and loneliness; and the built-in inequality of being secondary, which forces a secondary partner to agree to having less control over the terms and rules of the relationship.

Some people are able to tolerate the scarcity but not the the powerlessness, others are comfortable with giving up control but cannot accept the paucity of quality time and limits on frequency of contact. Many find it extremely difficult to accept either of these conditions, and chafe at the boundaries of a secondary relationship.

The poly community seems to be evenly divided on solutions to this dilemma. One school of thought says you will never be happy in this situation, as you are trying to have a primary relationship with someone who cannot provide the minimum amount of time and attention you need to feel safe and loved. This theory suggests that your only sane option is to get out now, as further misery awaits you if you continue to invest more time and energy in a losing proposition. The alternative idea is that you can stay in the relationship and work to create conditions that create an experience of greater safety and sufficiency for you. Only you can decide which strategy is best for you.

If you choose to stay with your partner, what can you do to improve your level of satisfaction and make peace with the situation? Three strategies have evolved which seem to work well for some people:

1) Seek out an additional relationship so that you are receiving more love and attention, in order to relieve the experience of scarcity and deprivation, or

2) Focus on creating your own full, exciting life separate from your partner, becoming more self-sufficient, so you will not be depending on your partner to give your life meaning and satisfaction, or

3) Develop a strong and trusting relationship with your partner and their primary partner, and explore ways to negotiate with them to enlarge the scope of the secondary relationship so you can get more of your needs met.

What if you choose to stay in your secondary relationship and look for another relationship? The goal can be to establish another secondary relationship to supplement what you are receiving in the current relationship, or to find a primary partner to more fully satisfy your need for commitment and companionship. Some people choose another secondary relationship so they can continue to prioritize the current relationship, be more available for that partner, and devote more energy to nurturing that relationship, as they have a high level of commitment and attachment to that partner. They identify the current relationship as primary even though their partner explicitly defines it as secondary. As a result, they prefer to hold onto the hope that this relationship will eventually be allowed to become primary, so they choose to get involved only in other secondary relationships.

Others choose to seek a primary relationship and gradually transfer their love and loyalty to that partner as the main object of their affection, as they realize that they need a primary relationship with more commitment, where they can have equal power rather than being limited by whatever rules their partner imposes. This can be a very painful transition, as it requires relinquishing the dream that the initial partner will make them primary, accepting that this is not likely to happen, and moving on to commit to a new partner who is more appropriate and available for a primary relationship.

Many secondary partners choose the second option, to stay in the relationship and become more self-sufficient. This allows them to enjoy and appreciate the love and companionship their partner is able to offer, while reducing the loneliness and resentments. There are many avenues to explore towards this goal, including making closer friendships, getting involved in activities you enjoy, investing more energy in your career or calling, or exploring a spiritual path. Any activity that makes you feel good about yourself and more fulfilled in other areas of your life is likely to make your relationship less critical to your well-being, and reduce your feelings of deprivation and mistreatment.

The most common strategy usually involves becoming more active in your community to create strong relationships with friends, family, co-workers, or activity partners. The more emotional intimacy and connection you can enjoy with others, the more satisfied you are likely to feel with your life. If more of your needs for companionship and community are met outside your romantic relationship, you are likely to feel less needy towards your partner. As a result you may feel more satisfied with the limited amount of time and commitment your partner can give you.

For example:

Jacob was in a secondary relationship with Rachel, but she was married to the rabbi of their reform synagogue. They were openly polyamorous, but Jacob felt snubbed at the synagogue because Rachel felt it was not appropriate to "flaunt" their relationship at services and events with their congregation. She was so busy with her husband and child that she had very little time for him. He felt especially lonely on all the Jewish holidays because he could not spend them with Rachel, and his family lived far away. Jacob decided to join a different synagogue, and became very involved with social activities there, volunteering for committees and facilitating groups and meetings. As he developed many close friends there and was invited to spend holidays at their homes, as well as feeling connected to people by attending services, he became more comfortable with the limits of his relationship with Rachel.

Rosa was involved in a secondary relationship with Jose, who lived with his primary partner, Leanna. Rosa was very lonely in the evenings and weekends, and her self-esteem plummeted because she felt abandoned by Jose and unimportant in his life. She was only allowed to see him one night a week. Jose spent the rest of his nights with Leanna, and on weekends he had custody of his two children from his previous relationship. Rosa decided to buy a condo, as she had been saving money for many years to become a homeowner. She was very proud of her achievement, as no one else in her family had ever owned their own home. She got very involved in fixing up her place, even taking classes on how to do home repairs. She took a real estate course and developed a strong friendship with a woman she met in the class. The two of them began a side-line business selling real estate, which became so successful that she quit her other job to pursue it full-time. A surprising side effect occurred: Jose was very impressed with the change in Rosa and was very proud of her achievements. He began to make himself more available, but ironically she had become so busy that she did not have much time for him. He courted her in earnest, pleading for more of her time and attention. She enjoyed this turn of events because previously she had always been feeling deprived and asking him for more.

The third strategy that works for some people is to work with your partner and their primary partner in the hopes of expanding the boundaries of your relationship, while still accepting that the relationship will be secondary. It is important to recognize that this is stressful and risky, and is not always possible. Two tasks are central to this strategy: identifying what is most important to you and will be likely to make you feel more satisfied in the relationship, and establishing a trusting enough relationship with both your partner and their primary partner to negotiate for whatever changes may be possible.

Think carefully about what components of a relationship are most important to your happiness, and make a list.

For some people, the central theme of this list is "More." You may want more time with your partner, more specific kinds of time such as on the weekends or holidays.

For example:

Janet and Joan had an agreement that they would only see outside partners on weeknights, and only two dates a month was the limit. Joan's secondary partner Linda, who felt starved for contact and affection, was able to negotiate with Janet to allow Joan to meet her for lunch and a walk once a week in between their dates, and that helped her feel much more satisfied without taking any time away from the primary relationship.

Or you may want more frequent contact, such as more phone calls or emails from your partner.

For example:

Paco found it difficult to feel connected to his partner Jessica because they lived in different cities and her husband Ricardo only felt comfortable with them meeting for dates once or twice a month. Paco was able to talk with both Jessica and Ricardo, and they agreed that Jessica would email him three or four times a week and that he could call her at work or at home as often as he wanted to, as long as he would accept it gracefully if she or Ricardo said it wasn't a good time to talk.

For others, the things they want the most involve expanding the limits prescribed by the primary relationship. This can cover a broad range of requests: wanting some public recognition as a partner, wanting to meet their partner's family, being included in special occasions and holidays, sharing possessions, being able to go away together for a weekend, or being allowed a fuller range of sexual activities.

For example:

Odessa wanted to host a birthday party at her home for her girlfriend Kate, but Kate's wife Jill felt threatened, as this was outside their agreement to keep their secondary relationships separate from their family and friends. With some negotiation, they were able to reach an agreement that Odessa and Jill would co-host the party.

Tanya is a bisexual woman in a secondary relationship with a bisexual man. She felt very hurt by the requirement that she and Malik use condoms for safer sex, as she felt she was being seen as a potential vector of disease. Malik and his primary partner Malcolm acknowledged that their safer sex rule had been imposed because their previous partners had been men, who have a relatively higher risk of STDs. They agreed to change the rule and allow Malik and Tanya to become fluid bonded and have unbarriered sex after all three were retested for HIV and other STDs, and had discussed their risk factors with their doctor.

Peter and Terese are a married couple; he fronts a punk rock band and she is their manager. Peter's secondary partner Sienna is a solo vocalist and she wanted to do a series of shows singing with Peter's band. She negotiated with Terese, who at first was uncomfortable with Sienna "invading" this area of their lives, as she felt this was "her turf." However, as a manager she could see that this would bring in a bigger audience and made good business sense, and that it would not change her relationship with Peter. This made Sienna much more satisfied with the secondary relationship because music was such a big part of her life that it had been very painful for her to be excluded from that whole arena of Peter's life.

Unfortunately, these happy endings tend to be the exception rather than the rule. Many people in secondary relationships make good faith efforts to create more space for an expanded relationship, but are unable to persuade their partner and/or their partner's primary partner to change the rules. Many polyamorous couples have set boundaries that work for them and are likely to see any proposed changes as a net loss to them and their relationship. In the above examples, expanded boundaries were possible because all partners could see some benefit in making the change, or at the very least the changes were experienced as "neutral" in that no one experienced significant loss of time, attention, or status. These changes are most likely to work if all parties can see that there is "something in it" for them, so you will greatly increase your chances of success by proposing ideas that do not seem to take something valuable away from your partner's primary relationship.

Some secondary relationships eventually start to turn into primary relationships, because people fall in love and develop much stronger attachments than originally planned. When this happens, it usually triggers feelings of fear and betrayal for the existing primary partner. They were promised that this wouldn't happen and that the secondary relationship would not become so important, but it did. Usually this happens over a long period of time when secondary relationships have time to grow and deepen, and it is usually not intentional. Often the importance of the secondary relationship begins to approach the level of love and commitment that exists in the primary relationship, creating confusion about the heirarchy of relationships. This usually precipitates a very messy relationship crisis which is best resolved through individual counseling and couples' counseling.

For example:

Tyrone and Andrea were a married couple. Tyrone had a secondary relationship with Missy which became much more serious over a two-year period. Tyrone and Missy both wanted to spend more time together, to become more public with their relationship, and to spend some holidays together. Tyrone approached Andrea to ask if she would be comfortable with his relationship with Missy becoming primary. At that point, five options were possible:

- The primary relationship between Tyrone and Andrea retains its status as the only primary relationship, and his relationship with Missy transitions back to being secondary, but with somewhat expanded boundaries.

- Missy does not accept being demoted back to a secondary status, and decides to leave the relationship.

- Both relationships become primary and a new set of guidelines is developed. This option can stipulate that both relationships are considered equally primary, or can delineate the relationship with Andrea as "more" primary. This relationship may have "seniority" in a number of ways, such as living together, owning property together, spending more time together, being connected to each other's families, etc.

- Andrea does not accept the secondary relationship becoming primary, and opts to leave the relationship and divorce Tyrone.

- Tyrone decides to leave Andrea for Missy. This may happen because he has gradually begun to feel closer to and more committed to Missy and feel ready to leave his marriage. However it may also have grown out of mistaken beliefs about the nature of long-term relationships and the illusion that the "grass is greener on the other side of the fence." It is extremely difficult for anyone to predict whether they will be happier by changing partners, and some people have regretted that decision.

If both relationships become primary, all three people must be able to successfully manage the transition. This requires a high degree of maturity, love, and highly developed interpersonal skills. Each partner has to stretch themselves and their boundaries to try to accommodate the needs of the other two people, while at the same time each sticking to their own bottom line and not agreeing to anything that will make them miserable. Many people have found this path extremely challenging and have eventually chosen other options. Often, one partner will eventually find this situation intolerable, and will either give their partner an ultimatum or opt out of the relationship.

As you can see, there is no easy or painless solution when one partner wants more is allowed by the limits of a secondary relationship. It is highly recommended that you seek individual or couples' counseling to help you decide how to proceed, as this can help you clarify your needs and explore what options are possible.

16
Women and Open Relationships: A Feminist Perspective

Many people have noticed that more men than women seem interested in open relationships. In most heterosexual relationships, it is the man who suggests polyamory to his spouse, or who insists on having outside partners. This trend has led many women to be suspicious of, or hostile to, this type of relationship.

Many women have viewed this issue through the lens of the historical oppression of women. As a result, they have seen polyamory as indistinguishable from polygamy or other relationship forms where men have multiple wives, concubines, "mistresses" or extramarital partners without the women's consent.

It has been accurately pointed out that in most societies which condone men having multiple wives and partners, women are treated as second-class citizens, often with few or no legal or political rights. In fact, in most cultures where women have finally won some amount of legal equality and political power, they have moved decisively to outlaw polygamy and to insist on monogamous relationships. As a result, having the power to demand monogamy from men has been seen by many feminists as evidence of women's progress towards equality.

In the past, a woman's body was viewed as the property of her husband, and her sexuality was considered subordinate to his sexual needs. She was likely to be emotionally and economically dependent on her partner. and to make her marriage central to her life. Even in most contemporary relationships, women tend to invest most of their emotional energy in the relationship and make it central in their lives. Many women struggle to maintain their independence and to achieve some semblance of equality in the relationship.

Polyamory Is Not the Same As Polygamy

However, polyamory is very different from past systems in two key components. First of all, in polygamous societies or other cultures where men have multiple wives or partners, men have the political and economic power to impose these relationships and women have no choice but to accept this arrangement. Secondly, while the men have many partners, the sexual double standard requires women to be monogamous and prevents them from enjoying the sexual and relationship freedom available to men.

In open relationships or polyamory, on the other hand, women have the power to negotiate the terms of the relationships, and to end the relationship if they do not want to consent to the man's demands. And women are equally free to pursue outside partners themselves. A crucial cornerstone of polyamory is a single standard of sexual behavior which allows men and women both to have multiple partners. Honesty, disclosure, and consent are the basic requirements of open relationships.

Some women advocate open relationships as a way to free women from the constraints of monogamy, giving them sexual freedom as well as independence from men. How can this be? In an open relationship, a woman's body and her sexuality belong to her, not to her male partner, and she can freely choose her sexual partners. Likewise, she can have more than one intimate relationship, and can have more than one source of closeness and emotional support. As a result, she is likely to be less dependent on a husband or male partner for love, intimacy, sex, and companionship.

Some women feel that an open relationship gives a woman much more control over her own life, as she has the power to make decisions about how to organize her time, her priorities, and her family life. Some polyamorous women believe they are less vulnerable to being controlled by any one man, as they have more independence from one man's influence in their lives. And having the option of more than one relationship means they do not have to settle for an unsatisfactory relationship. Being in an open relationship gives some women more bargaining power to ask for what they want and to create a level playing field.

Some women have conceptualized polyamory as part of their feminist ideology, seeing it as a manifestation of the feminist slogan that "the personal is political."

For example:

Betsy is a 54-year-old schoolteacher whose two grown daughters were scandalized by their mother's polyamorous lifestyle. They said they were embarrassed to bring the grandchildren to her home because she lived openly with her two lovers, a man and a woman. She wrote them a letter explaining, "I am a veteran of more than forty years of activism in the women's movement. In the 1960s, we fought for women's right to access to birth control, so we could take control our own sexuality for the first time in history and decide when and if to get pregnant. In the 1970s, I worked for women's right to choose abortion, to control our own bodies and decide whether to bear a child or not. In the 1980s, I worked at a rape crisis center to fight for women's right to be free from violence and say no to rape and unwanted sexual harassment, to demand the right to control who we have sex with. Since the 1990s I have been in a polyamorous relationship because I own my own sexuality and I can choose who to have sex with and who to be in a relationship with, and what the rules of my relationships will be. This is at the core of feminism: the right to control our bodies and our sexuality. No man can own me or control my body. My sexuality belongs to me and I have the power to decide how to express it and with whom."

What If a Man Pressures a Woman Into Polyamory?

While many women praise the liberating empowerment of open relationships, some experience a much different reality. Many women who have been in monogamous relationships or marriages feel coerced into polyamory when their partner or husband starts an outside relationship and insists that they accept it. Polyamory by definition involves the consent of all parties and should not be forced on a partner against her will.

While the feminist movement has dramatically changed our world to create many more rights and opportunities for women, some women still feel powerless in relationships with men. Many factors contribute to this inequality. We are socialized as women to accept the authority of men and defer to a male partner. In addition, women still make a lot less money than men, and many women leave the paid labor force for years to raise children, effectively lowering their salaries and undermining their career success. As a result, many women are emotionally and economically dependent on their male partner and do not have equal power in the relationship. Thus, when a man arbitrarily changes the rules in a monogamous relationship by becoming sexually involved with another woman or man, his wife or primary partner is often in a weakened position and feels compelled to accept it against her will.

For example:

Rosanna, a 35-year-old wife and mother, said, "I had just had our second child and had taken a year off to stay home so I could breastfeed the new baby, so I was at home with an infant and a toddler. My employer laid me off because I was taking more time off than the maximum that they were required to allow. I lost my health insurance and was dependent, not only on my husband's income to support our whole family, but also on the health insurance we got through his job. He announced that he wanted an open relationship and that he was already sleeping with a woman he worked with and wanted to have an ongoing relationship with her. I told him I didn't want that, but he refused to consider ending this other relationship. I considered separation or divorce, but I would have been out in the cold with no job, no income, and no health insurance, a single mother raising two kids on my own. I felt trapped but I had no choice."

Patsy was irate that her husband Finn read about polyamory on-line and decided he wanted to try it. She tried to insist on keeping the monogamous relationship which they had agreed to when they got married ten years before. He refused, admitting that he had already had two affairs and that he would continue to have sex with other women.

She felt she had no choice but to stay in the marriage and accept Finn's sexual relationships with other women, while she remained monogamous.

Tanya says bluntly, "How is polyamory any different from what women have always had to put up with? My mother tolerated my father's affairs for thirty years because she got married when she was 18 and had never had a job outside the home, and couldn't survive financially without him. My grandmother went through the same thing with an alcoholic husband who slept around whenever he was drinking. Now my husband is trying to force me to accept the same old shit with a fancy new name." She divorced her husband Johann when he refused to end his outside relationships, but agonized over the decision because she knew that it would be very hard on their kids, and that the whole family would suffer financially from the divorce.

Lee-Ming came to the U.S. from China to go to medical school. She fell in love and married Feng, a fellow medical student, and they moved to a remote area in Montana to do their medical residency. Feng got involved with another woman and refused to stop seeing her, despite Lee-Ming's requests that he honor their monogamous marriage agreement. She knew if she divorced him and moved out she would have to drop out of her residency and would not be able to complete her requirements to become a doctor. In addition, she feared deportation, because they had only been married for one year and the INS was scrutinizing her citizenship. She felt stuck, and stayed in the marriage for three more years and tolerated her husband's affair under duress, until she was able to complete the residency, file for divorce, and move to another state where she could find a job.

Some people would argue that these examples are not actually polyamory, since in each case the woman has not given their consent and the man has imposed this unilaterally. However, I present these examples because such situations have served to alienate many women from the idea of open relationships. Of course there are comparable situations where a woman decides to become polyamorous and imposes this on her male partner without his consent, but this situation is much less common.

Some couples facing this situation have developed creative solutions. The man is asking his wife to accept something that he wants very much, to have an open relationship, something that she doesn't want and which is very difficult and painful for her. So I suggest that the woman ask the man to give her something that she really wants that is very difficult for him, in return for her acceptance of him having other partners.

For example:

Octavia decided to ask her husband Henry to support her financially to go back to school and complete her PhD, since she had to drop out several years previously while juggling two children and a full-time job. She understood that it would be difficult for their family to live on her husband's income alone, and that he would have to help more with housework and taking care of the children. She offered to accept his outside relationship, which was very painful for her, if he would agree to do this for her in exchange. It wasn't easy for either of them, but she spent the next two years finishing her dissertation and getting her doctorate, and he was allowed to continue his other relationship. They both stretched themselves to do something that was very challenging and their marriage survived and eventually even thrived.

Sarah and Joshua were living in New York City, on the verge of divorce because Joshua was having casual sexual relationships with many other women, but Sarah wanted a monogamous relationship. She hated living in the city and told him she would agree to a polyamorous marriage if he agreed that they could move to a less urban area. He loved the big city but agreed that if she could become more comfortable with an open relationship, he could be happy living in a small town in Connecticut that was still close enough to his job.

In each of these examples, it was important to the woman that the man recognize just how difficult it was for her to accept an open relationship. By agreeing to do something she wanted that was just as hard for him, he was giving the woman some power and making it more of a win-win situation. These women initially experience polyamory as a terrible loss, in that they are losing the exclusive relationship they previously had and losing control over the terms of their marriage. As a result, asking the husband for a meaningful concession allows them to gain something that is valuable to them and to feel more equal.

Why Do More Men Than Women Want Open Relationships?

Many have theorized about why so many more men than women are interested in open relationships. It may be more of a "public relations" issue than anything else. Because this type of relationship is most associated in the public imagination with sex and sexual variety rather than relationships and emotional intimacy, it attracts the attention of more men than women. Men have been trained and socialized to value sex very highly and to compartmentalize sex, separating sex from love. As a result, it is often easier for men to enjoy having more than one sexual partner.

Some scientists also believe that men are "wired" to crave many sexual partners because it serves an evolutionary purpose: the more women a man has sex with, the more women he may impregnate, and this encourages the survival of the species. So, says this theory, men are often drawn to polyamory for the allure of having many sex partners and enjoying lots of sex, more than for the promise of intimate relationships.

In addition, men's libidos seem to be heavily driven by novelty and sexual variety. They are often most attracted to the experience of sleeping with new and different sexual partners, and the novelty of someone new and unknown carries a very potent erotic charge in the male imagination.

Conversely, women are socialized to value relationships, companionship, and emotional intimacy over sex, and are taught that sex without love is immoral or devoid of meaning. For women, a new sexual partner may be intriguing, but may carry more dangers than it does for men. Women who have sex with a new man risk physical assault, robbery, rape, pregnancy, HIV/AIDS, and even murder, as they are putting themselves in a very vulnerable position with someone who they don't know very well and who is likely to be capable of physically overpowering them. With the increased anonymity of meeting partners over the Internet, the danger of violence and coercion has escalated. Many women have reported terrifying experiences, such as going on a date and being forced into sex without a condom, threatened and coerced into anal sex or some other sexual activity that was not agreed on, being beaten or stalked by men, being robbed and becoming victims of identity theft. Men who have sex with a number of women generally do not face such risks.

In addition, many women feel much more physically vulnerable during the act of sex than men do. Because intercourse requires a woman to allow a man to enter and penetrate her body, many women describe feeling much more emotionally vulnerable during sex than their male partners. As a result, the cost/benefit analysis for women is different than for men, and since the "cost" is so much higher, many women are much more reluctant than men to have outside sexual partners, and are much more selective about who they sleep with and under what circumstances.

The Double Standard and Polyamory

Another less tangible factor inhibits women from being polyamorous. Many women believe that even though their male partners have outside relationships, that a double standard still exists both in society and in their relationship. They fear that their husbands or male partners are comfortable having sex with other women, but will be angry and lose respect for them if they do likewise. In some cases this fear has turned out to be well founded.

For example:

Doreen reported that her husband Hal slept with many women, but whenever she wanted to have an outside partner, Hal found some reason to object to the potential partner, becoming angry and withdrawn if she started to date anyone.

Patty explained that her husband Paul had two ongoing secondary relationships with other women. However, he was crushed after she slept with someone else for the first time and refused to have sex with her for several months. Paul said, "When Patty has sex with another man, I feel that it 'cheapens' our sexual relationship — I can't the same way about her, knowing that she had had sex with someone else." Patty felt punished by Paul for being polyamorous, while Paul was allowed to continue having two other relationships.

Many men who thought they wanted an open relationship, and who enjoy having other partners, are surprised to discover that they are not comfortable with their wives having sex or a relationship with another man. Part of this experience is just the normal jealousy experienced in any open relationship, but many men find that there is something deeper, an ingrained belief that a woman should be "faithful" and that it is "wrong" for a woman to stray outside the primary relationship. Some men have been surprised that they still harbor some remnants of the belief that women are either "madonnas" or "whores," and if their partner sleeps with someone else, she moves from the madonna category to the whore category in their minds.

It is important to be compassionate with ourselves and our partners in such situations, because we have been heavily socialized by society and religion to believe that a woman who is not sexually exclusive with her husband or male partner is immoral and worthy of contempt. These misogynist attitudes about women's sexuality are deeply entrenched in our culture, and require discussion, education, and effort to dislodge and replace with more egalitarian, sex-positive beliefs. Some men, through much personal growth work in therapy or through internal soul-searching, are able to let go of this sexist programming and to accept that their partner can have outside partners without being knocked off the pedestal on which they have unfortunately placed her. Luckily these attitudes are less pronounced in those of younger generations who were raised in a more open and feminist era with accurate sex education and less rigid gender roles.

I encourage couples to talk through their feelings, either on their own or with a couples counselor, to identify residual attitudes that may need adjusting. It is sometimes difficult to differentiate between normal jealousy and sexist programming, and this process can require some internal work or counseling to unpack and change.

What's In It for Women? More Love and Emotional Connection!

On the positive side, more women are learning that polyamory is not just about sex, and can include having more than one loving, intimate relationship. This holds much more appeal for a broader cross-section of women, as many women are not satisfied with the amount of intimacy, closeness, and companionship they receive in their primary relationship. While many men may be motivated to seek outside partners because they want more sex and sexual variety, women are more likely to be seeking intimacy, time, and romantic attention from an outside relationship.

For many women, the most important selling point for an open relationship is the promise of more love and emotional connection. It is not exactly news that many women experience a longing for more intimacy than their male partner can provide, and report feeling lonely and chronically deprived of attention and emotional connection. As a result, having outside relationships with other partners can go a long way towards a feeling of satisfaction and an abundance of love.

For example:

Billie described always feeling there was a shortage of attention and emotional support from her husband, constantly asking him for more closeness and affection. After initiating an open relationship and dating other men, she said, "For the first time in my life, I have enough of everything and don't feel starved!"

Meg said, "This is the truly revolutionary thing about polyamory. A woman can feel safe asking for what she wants and not having to settle for less. I can have my needs met for love and intimacy, and feel truly satisfied."

Paradoxically, the fact that so many women feel dissatisfied with their relationship in the first place is often the key reason they feel reluctant to consent to their husband's request for an open relationship.

For example:

Jessica felt like she wasn't getting enough time, love, and attention from her partner Adam, and felt sure that if he got involved with other women that she would receive even less. However, when she started dating other people, she found herself showered with romantic attention, affection, companionship, and quality time with other partners. And the fact that so many men were asking her out made Adam appreciate her more and become much more attentive .

There is no right or wrong answer about whether polyamory is better or worse for women than monogamy. Some women need and want a monogamous relationship, and others are much happier in an open relationship. What is clear is that women must work to achieve equal power in relationships with men in order to effectively negotiate for the type of relationship that is right for them. It is the power imbalance rather than polyamory or monogamy that is the problem, because it denies women the choice. Coercion is not the same as consent, whether to polyamory or to monogamy.

LOVE IN ABUNDANCE

CONCLUSION AND RESOURCE LIST

Conclusion: A Few Parting Words on Healthy, Happy, Sustainable Open Relationships

Because I am a counselor, I work with people every day who are facing some challenges with open relationships. As a result, most of this book is focused on the most common problems you may encounter and techniques for resolving them. While no relationship is free of conflicts and challenges, polyamorous relationships have some very different features and parameters than monogamous relationships. As a result, the kinds of problems most likely to occur in polyamorous relationships require their own unique solutions, which I have tried to provide in this book.

Although this book is primarily focused on problem-solving, that is not meant to imply that polyamorous relationships are filled with conflict, angst, and drama. Don't be discouraged by reading about all the potential difficulties faced by people in this lifestyle. I have presented so many examples of "poly blunders" in the hopes that you can learn from their mistakes and prevent problems before they start. Open relationships are no more problematic than monogamous relationships, and many people have created healthy and happy long-term polyamorous relationships. Like any successful relationship, an open relationship requires commitment, effort, integrity, honesty, and maturity.

Your chances of success can be dramatically improved by utilizing the resources which now exist. Over the past decade, websites, support groups, workshops, and books about polyamory have become widely available for the first time. There are now counselors with expertise on open relationships, while in the past most therapists pathologized polyamory and insisted that their clients return to a monogamous relationship. There are even attorneys that assist polyamorous couples and families in protecting themselves, their assets, and their children. These resources offer a "safety net" of support and community which help strengthen and enhance polyamorous relationships.

In addition, more polyamorous people have "come out of the closet" and are now having multiple relationships openly, rather than hiding behind the public facade of monogamous relationships. Some groups have worked very hard to educate the public and to organize politically to advocate for societal acceptance of open relationships, as well as for legal rights and recognition of such relationships. These changes have created a climate of greater public understanding of open relationships and a safer environment for more people to make the decision to explore this lifestyle. The Internet has made it much easier for people who desire open relationships to access information and education, to meet other people who share their orientation, and to create relationships.

Very little research has been done on people in open relationships, so no one really knows how prevalent this relationship orientation is nor how many people practice this type of relationship. No statistics exist on what percentage of couples are polyamorous, nor how many of these are successful in the long run. There are a number of small research projects currently being conducted by social scientists, but it will probably be years before they will be able to provide much useful data. In the meantime, I can offer only anecdotal evidence. In my personal life and my professional work, I have met or spoken with hundreds of people who have successfully established long-term open relationships. Through my professional network, I have been told about hundreds more, who I have not met personally but who are happily engaged in healthy polyamorous relationships. While this is no substitute for rigorous scientific study, no hard numbers currently exist.

This dearth of data should not be a deterrent to those who would like to explore this option of experiencing multiple relationships. Pioneers have always had to venture into unknown territory armed with the right tools and with faith in themselves. They must feel that the benefits they hope to achieve will outweigh the risks they are undertaking. For those who succeed in polyamory, the rewards are significant. Open relationships can provide an abundance of love far beyond what most people have experienced. To be held in the heart of one spouse or lover is sublime, and to experience intimacy with more than one partner can be exponentially satisfying. Having the support, companionship, and love of multiple partners can enrich and expand our experience of love, family, and community. It can also engender deep personal growth which can strengthen each individual and enhance our happiness and quality of life. I would encourage anyone who feels drawn to this orientation to start by taking small steps on this path and proceed slowly but surely, seeking the help and support you need at each step of the way. If you think each step through and practice this lifestyle mindfully and with integrity, you will have no regrets.

Appendix: More Resources On Open Relationships

Just a few short years ago, there were very few books or other resources available to people trying to learn about and practice polyamory. Luckily, in the past decade, a number of excellent books and articles have been written and there are numerous websites devoted to this increasingly popular subject. In addition there are conferences, workshops, classes, and podcasts on open relationships. Accessing some of these resources can accelerate your learning curve and help you avoid or solve the many challenges that can arise, whichever form of polyamorous relationships you choose.

Books on polyamory

The Ethical Slut: A Practical Guide to Polyamory, Open Relationships, and Other Adventures, by Dossie Easton and Janet W. Hardy, Second Edition, Ten Speed Press, 2009

Polyamory: The New Love Without Limits, by Deborah M. Anapol, Intinet Resource Center, 1997

The Lesbian Polyamory Reader: Open Relationships, Non-Monogamy, and Casual Sex, edited by Marcia Munson and Judith P. Stelboum, Haworth Press, 1999

Lesbian Polyfidelily: A Pleasure Guide for All Women Whose Hearts are Open to Multiple Sexualoves, by Celeste West, Booklegger Publishing, 1996

Redefining Our Relationships: Guidelines for Responsible Open Relationships, by Wendy-O Matik, Defiant Times Press, 2002

Opening Up: A Guide to Creating and Sustaining Open Relationships, by Tristan Taormino, Cleis Press, 2008

Open: Love, Sex, and Life in an Open Marriage, by Jenny Block, Avalon Publishing, 2008

The Poly Communication Survival Kit, by Robert McGarey, 1992. This book is out of print but is available in PDF format for download at www.HumanPotentialCenter.org/Poly

Periodicals on Polyamory

Loving More Magazine, on-line and in print magazine on open relationships, available at www.lovemore.com or through Loving More Foundation, (303)-543-7540

Books on Jealousy

Romantic Jealousy: Causes, Symptoms, and Cures, by Ayala Pines, St. Martin's Press, 1996

Romantic Jealousy: Understanding and Conquering the Shadow of Love, by Ayala Pines, St. Martin's Press, 1992

The Green-Eyed Marriage: Surviving Jealous Relationships, by Robert Barker, The Free Press, 1987

Jealousy, by Nancy Friday, Bantam, 1987

Jealousy, by Gordon Clanton and Lynn G. Smith, University Press of America, 1986

Jealousy: Experiences and Solutions, by Hildegard Baumgart, University of Chicago Press, 1990

The Psychology of Jealousy and Envy, by Peter Salovey, Ed; Guilford Press, 1991

Excellent article on jealousy by Ralph B. Hupka: "Cultural Determinants of Romantic Jealousy," in *Alternative Lifestyles* Volume 4, 1981

Other resources: workshops, classes, and coaching on open relationships:

Loving More (national conferences, workshops, etc), www. lovemore.com or (303)-543-7540

World Polyamory Association, www.worldypolyamoryassociation. org, or (808) 244-4103

Wendy-O Matik (workshops and classes), www.wendyomatik.com

Reid Mihalko and LiYana Silver, wwwReidAboutSex.com or (917)- 207-4554

Dawn Davidson and Akien McLean, Mandala Enterprises, www. weirdness.org or www.mandalaenterprises.com

Kathy Labriola, (51 0)-84 1-5307 or anarchofeminist@yahoo.com

To find a therapist or couples counselor with expertise on open relationships:

The Poly-Friendly Professionals Directory: www.polychromatic. com/pfp

Kink-Aware Professionals Network: www.kinkawareprofessionals.org

Loving More Poly Professionals Listings: www.lovemore.com/ polyprofessional.html

New Monogamy: Redifining Relationship After
Fidelity
- infedelity
- stages of recovery
  → crisis
  → understanding/insight phase
  → vision phase
- both partners are to blame.
- one couple can go through several different
  marriages
  → newly weds, career, family, post-career,
    post-family
- causes: child birth.
- implicits become explicits

- not talking about
  what we believe to
  be traditional
  marriages.

The Chronological of Water
- Sex Surrogate - in place of partner
  → The Sessions - movie
- substance abuse, marriage, child abuse, grief
- triggering - birthing a dead child - vaginal birth -
  38 hrs.
- serious substance abuse issues - not about recovery/
  sobriety.
- flunks out - abuses boyfriend -

Adjustment
Disorder

The Monster Under The Bed
- self help style book
- put off talking about things like sex
- Sex was blown off
  → nobody talked about new anti-depressients lower libido
- Doctors only have 10 hrs of sexual education.

Intimacy from the Inside Out - JoEllen Notte
- working for his own marriage
- 1/2 year training - 3 days a week
- training - social justice need

About the Author

Kathy Labriola is a nurse, counselor, and hypnotherapist in private practice in Berkeley, California. She has been a card-carrying bisexual and polyamorist for nearly 40 years. She is political activist and community organizer, rides a bike, and raises chickens and organic vegetables in her back yard. She can be reached at anarchofeminist@yahoo.com.

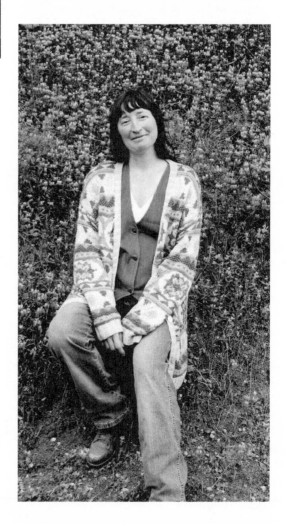

GENERAL SEXUALITY

A Hand In the Bush: The Fine Art of Vaginal Fisting
Deborah Addington $13.95

The Lazy Crossdresser
Charles Anders $13.95

Phone Sex: Oral Skills and Aural Thrills
Miranda Austin $15.95

Sex Disasters... And How to Survive Them
C. Moser, Ph.D., M.D. & Janet W. Hardy $16.95

Tricks... To Please a Man
Tricks... To Please a Woman
both by Jay Wiseman $13.95 ea.

When Someone You Love Is Kinky
Dossie Easton & Catherine A. Liszt $15.95

BDSM/KINK

At Her Feet: Powering Your Femdom Relationship *(fall 2010)*
TammyJo Eckhart & Fox $14.95

... But I Know What You Want: 25 Sex Tales for the Different
James Williams $13.95

The Compleat Spanker
Lady Green $12.95

Conquer Me: girl-to-girl wisdom about fulfilling your submissive desires
Kacie Cunningham $13.95

Erotic Slavehood: A Miss Abernathy Omnibus
Christina Abernathy $15.95

Family Jewels: A Guide to Male Genital Play and Torment
Hardy Haberman $12.95

Flogging
Joseph W. Bean $12.95

The Human Pony: A Guide for Owners, Trainers and Admirers
Rebecca Wilcox $27.95

Intimate Invasions: The Ins and Outs of Erotic Enema Play
M.R. Strict $13.95

The Kinky Girl's Guide to Dating
Luna Grey $16.95

The Mistress Manual: A Good Girl's Guide to Female Dominance
Mistress Lorelei $16.95

The New Bottoming Book
The New Topping Book
Dossie Easton & Janet W. Hardy $14.95 ea.

The (New and Improved) Loving Dominant
John and Libby Warren $16.95

Play Piercing
Deborah Addington $13.95

Radical Ecstasy: SM Journeys to Transcendence
Dossie Easton & Janet W. Hardy $16.95

The Seductive Art of Japanese Bondage
Midori, photographs by Craig Morey $27.95

The Sexually Dominant Woman: A Workbook for Nervous Beginners
Lady Green $11.95

SM 101: A Realistic Introduction
Jay Wiseman $24.95

21st Century Kinkycrafts
edited by Janet Hardy $19.95

TOYBAG GUIDES:
A Workshop In A Book   **$9.95 each**

Age Play, by Bridgett "Lee" Harrington

Basic Bondage, by Jay Wiseman *(fall 2010)*

Canes and Caning, by Janet W. Hardy

Clips and Clamps, by Jack Rinella

Dungeon Emergencies & Supplies, by Jay Wiseman

Erotic Knifeplay, by Miranda Austin & Sam Atwood

Foot and Shoe Worship, by Midori

High-Tech Toys, by John Warren

Hot Wax and Temperature Play, by Spectrum

Medical Play, by Tempest

Playing With Taboo, by Mollena Williams

Greenery Press books are available from your favorite on-line or brick-and-mortar bookstore or erotic boutique, or direct from The Stockroom, www.stockroom.com, 1-800-755-TOYS.